Praise for *Meditation for Life*

"*Justyn Comer's Meditation for Life is the best introduction I have come across to a practice that can profoundly improve one's life personally and professionally. As a psychiatrist, this book will be an invaluable resource to my patients, friends, and colleagues.*"

J. Andrew Huchingson MD. *Board Certified Adult Psychiatrist, Assistant Clinical Professor. Medical University of South Carolina*

"*Comer writes with a dry, self-deprecating wit that disguises his great spiritual wisdom; this is a funny book that only later did I realize was deeply serious. Avoiding completely the mumbo jumbo language that made me skeptical of meditation, Comer introduces us to a simple, effective, and worthwhile practice that delivers immediate, obvious results. I don't usually like people getting in my head, but reading this book, I'm happy to make an exception.*"

M.A.Wallace, *Writer, New York City*

"*This is a thorough, brilliant, and compelling introduction to the practice of meditation. Each chapter examines a critical facet of the practice opening the reader to its powerful benefits. I found, after completing each chapter, I simply could not wait to begin and try it that day. It is as if Mr. Comer was reading my mind, helping me to proceed through the next step. This is a simply marvelous introduction to a whole new awareness and ignites a strong desire to meditate daily, making it a joy and giving the reader competence and confidence.*"

Reverend Janet Broderick, *Rector, St. Peter's Episcopal Church, Morristown, New Jersey*

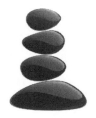

MEDITATION
FOR LIFE

How mind training improves
relationships, career, health and happiness

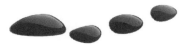

JUSTYN COMER

MEDITATION FOR LIFE

How mind training improves relationships, career, health and happiness

First published in 2018 by
Panoma Press Ltd
48 St Vincent Drive, St Albans, Herts, AL1 5SJ UK

info@panomapress.com
www.panomapress.com

Cover design by Michael Inns
Artwork by Karen Gladwell

ISBN 978-1-784521-23-3

Contents

Introduction

'… and what do you do for a living?'

I used to have an easy answer to this question. I told people I worked on Wall Street, or that I was a management consultant. People were comfortable with these conventional, to-be-expected answers. We may not have had anything in common yet, but we knew how to continue our conversation.

Today, however, I pause before answering. I pause because I know that my response will be either a conversation-starter or a complete conversation-stopper.

'Errr … I teach meditation.'

Then I watch for their reaction.

Sometimes people freeze for a second before looking around the room for someone else to talk to. Oh, well.

There is, however, another common reaction.

'Wow! I wish I could do that. I never could though. I can't sit still for a moment, and my mind's all over the place.'

Of the two reactions, this one bothers me more. It bothers me because it means this person genuinely believes meditation is not for them. They imagine that people who meditate have some kind of superhuman ability to calm their minds and sit in peaceful bliss with perfect concentration. They think they lack the skills necessary to meditate because their mind is *'all over the place.'* Unfortunately, many people believe the same thing.

This belief is wrong.

Everybody's minds are all over the place.

We meditate *because* our minds are all over the place.

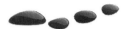

I was eight years old when I was first introduced to the tricky nature of mind. My history teacher, Mr. Hicks, gave us a challenge. 'Try,' he instructed the class, *'not* to think about pink elephants.' Now, since I can't work out the relationship between this exercise and history, I imagine we were being particularly difficult, and he was attempting to settle us down.

Try it yourself, right now. *Don't think about pink elephants.*

Impossible, isn't it? By following the instruction, we're forced to imagine pink elephants so that we know what not to think about. But the moment we're thinking about pink elephants, *we're thinking about pink elephants!*

The only way not to think of pink elephants is to forget about the challenge altogether. Then we will not be thinking about pink elephants, but nor will we be thinking about the challenge, which means we haven't solved anything…

The pink elephant problem kept my class amused – possibly even quiet – for a few minutes.

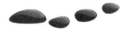

In introductory meditation classes, I don't ask people not to think about pink elephants. But I ask them to do something almost as frustrating. I ask them to hold their attention on their breathing; to notice their breath as it comes in and as it goes out.

Most people manage for a few seconds before their minds wander off in random directions. Some start to wonder whether they're doing it right, or how this focus on breathing could possibly be useful. Others remember that they forgot to feed the dog. They start worrying about who's going to pick up the kids from school, or whether it's going to rain and, if it is, whether they've got the umbrella. They get distracted.

They're not the only ones.

My mind wanders off in various directions as well. One place it likes to go is to analyze recent conversations. I start wondering,

"What really happened there?"

"Did I misunderstand them? Could I have been misunderstood?"

"I should have said [x, y, or z] which would have been so much cleverer."

Another place it likes to go is to try to solve problems. Anything that's even slightly unresolved in my life pops into my head. I start thinking about finances, family issues, or how I'm going to write the next chapter of this book.

Sometimes my mind starts daydreaming about random things like whether my soccer team can win the league this year, or how one day I'd like to visit Vancouver.

My point is that I've been meditating for over thirty years, but my mind is probably quite similar to yours. I point it in a direction such as focusing on the breath – and then it wanders.

Zen teacher Thich Nhat Hanh illustrates our relationship with our minds via the story of a man on a horse. "The horse is galloping quickly. It appears that the man is going somewhere important. Another man, standing alongside the road, shouts: 'Where are you going?' The man on the horse replies, 'I don't know! Ask the horse!' "

This is the first insight of meditation: *We're not as in control of our minds as we think.* We may like to believe that we choose where our minds go, but as soon as we start meditating, we discover that our minds are like the horse. We are the rider. We go where our minds lead us. Not the other way around.

If you have a sense that your mind is all over the place, welcome to being human! Minds wander. It's what they do. You might think your mind is particularly frantic, but that's because you can't see inside everyone else's minds and recognize that they are equally distracted. People are like you. They may appear to be normal and together. But their minds are all over the place as well.

Take a breath. Not metaphorically. Literally: take a breath. Now.

Notice the air as it comes in and goes out.

If you managed that, you can meditate. We'll get into the details later but, for now, please believe that if you can breathe, you can do this. Yes, your mind wanders. So does mine. So does everyone's. It doesn't mean you can't meditate. It means you're normal.

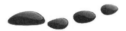

Luckily for me, I discovered meditation when I was too young to worry about whether I could do it or not. I was fourteen when a Christian priest introduced me to a basic practice as part of training for Confirmation. Since then, I've studied at Buddhist monasteries in India, Europe, and the United States. At university, I did a degree in Theology and Religious Studies and meditated using a technique from the Hindu tradition. I've practiced with Christian contemplatives and explored the approaches of non-religious meditation organizations, such as Jon Kabat-Zinn's Center for Mindfulness.

The main influence for my practice and teaching was a small meditation community I belonged to in the 1990s. We had an eclectic teacher who borrowed from several traditions; primarily Zen and Tibetan Buddhism.

We were a serious spiritual group, using meditation as our primary discipline. Sometimes we would do long stints as a group for several hours. Most of the time we were on our own doing two one-hour sessions per day. However, even when we were not 'meditating' we were still practicing.

We didn't live in a monastery. We lived in the real world, had jobs, families, and friends. Nevertheless, no matter what we were doing, whether it was laundry, going for a run or giving a corporate presentation, we were taught to hold our attention with the same degree of focus as if we were meditating. We used every moment as an opportunity to develop spiritual insight and growth.

Everything we did was used to help our meditation practice. What we quickly noticed, however, was that our meditation practice helped everything we did. The level and quality of our practice showed up in our lives. When we were diligent in our practice, our work, relationships, health, and happiness, were all enhanced.

In 1997 our teacher invited us to start teaching in public. It took me a couple of years to get started, but eventually, I decided to focus my teaching on this practical aspect of meditation – that it improves everyday life. I could have focused on the spiritual aspect, but I saw so many people who were missing out on the numerous benefits of meditation because they had no interest in spirituality or religion.

If I have a 'thing' that defines my teaching, it is this:

Meditation can help every aspect of your life.

Career, relationships, health, happiness, athletics, art, creativity, or anything else you'd like to improve: all are enhanced by the practice of meditation.

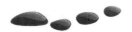

Coverage of meditation has exploded over recent years. Like most long-term meditators, I'm delighted that everyone has now heard about it. I have nevertheless been disappointed at how narrowly it tends to be portrayed. Most people still regard it either as a spiritual exercise or as a relaxation technique. It can be those things. But it is so much more.

This book is my attempt to explain what else is on offer.

Book Structure

The beginning, middle, and end of this book are really three sections: the *what,* the *why,* and the *how* of meditation.

Chapter 1 is my attempt at explaining *what* meditation is.

Chapters 2 through 6 offer various reasons *why* you should meditate. This is not exhaustive. Meditation helps more than what is listed here, but these chapters cover four of the main aspects of people's lives: relationships, career, health, and happiness.

Chapters 7 and 8 give guidance on *how* to meditate.

The chapters build on each other but are also intended to be self-contained, so that if you are only interested in health or in happiness, you can skip there. Nevertheless, I'd suggest you at least give the first chapter a quick read, so you understand where I'm coming from.

My goal is to inspire you to see meditation as more than a religious discipline or stress relief. I want you to see it can be a powerful tool for all aspects of your life. If you used to meditate, but have stopped, I hope you find the inspiration to get back to it. If you've never meditated, I hope you will start.

What is Meditation?

A few years back, I went on a tour around Burgundy in France. In one sense Burgundy is a relatively small and straightforward wine region. It is known for one white wine (Chardonnay), one red (Pinot Noir), and grows almost nothing else.

I had expected to see opulent estates like the ones in Bordeaux, but Burgundy is more modest and feels like a simple farming community. Basically, there's a single main road running North–South with grapevines on either side. Every few miles there's a little village, and that's about it.

The tour started in the region's unofficial capital, Beaune. Initially, our guide, Florian, took us north to visit wineries famous for Pinot Noir, and then we headed south for lunch in Montrachet, renowned for Chardonnay. In the afternoon, we stopped at various vineyards on the way back to where we had started. It was a wonderful day, we learned a great deal, and all the wines we tasted were incredible.

Over the course of the tour, we learned that there is a great deal of complexity in sub-categories of the two wines produced. We learned that grapes from east of the road are made into generic Burgundy wine. Wine from grapes to the west of the road is more complicated. To start with the wine gets a different title, named after the village it comes from. Wine from specific plots will, in turn, have the name of the field specified on the label. Within each field, every three rows of vines can have different owners, who will grow the grapes differently, make the wine their own way, and get their own name on the label. As a result, the very small area that is Burgundy, only making two types of wine, actually produces thousands of slightly different wines.

When I'm asked, *'What is meditation?'* I feel it's like trying to describe Burgundy. The answer is both simple, and at the same time surprisingly complex. In one sense meditation covers a relatively small area of human activity. But, like Burgundy, within that small area, there are numerous techniques and countless nuances.

We could have gone on a tour of Burgundy with someone other than Florian. It might have been wonderful, and it might have been similar, but it would have been different. Another guide would have taken us to different wineries; they would have had different interests; and would have told different stories. Most tours are done in buses, but Florian is passionate about the outdoors, so he runs his tours using bicycles. On another tour, Burgundy would still have been Burgundy, but our tour was uniquely Florian's.

Different meditation teachers emphasize different aspects of meditation. Some will focus on a specific technique, looking at the emotional or spiritual benefits that come with it. Others may approach meditation from a religious or cultural point of view putting it within an ethical or metaphysical context. Some teachers are using meditation to achieve certain specific outcomes such as improved concentration, relaxation, or focus, and will group a number of techniques based on their objectives. I don't think any of them are wrong for teaching it the way they do, and I am not right for presenting it the way I do. Like Florian, I am going to present my view of meditation which is a reflection of my interests, my experiences and what I've found to be helpful for me. It's not the only way; it's just mine.

Nor am I going to present all of meditation here. Florian showed us a great deal of Burgundy in a day, but if we had been there for a month, there would still have been more to discover. Likewise, there is more to meditation than I could cover in a thousand pages. Florian inspired us to appreciate and try the wines, knowing that we could then continue to deepen our relationship with Burgundy wines for the rest of our lives. I also hope to inspire you to understand what is available from meditating, to encourage you to try it, and then for you to continue to explore it on your own. There will always be more to discover.

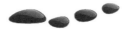

At a high level, there are two wines in Burgundy, and I suggest there are three reasons to meditate: to feel better, to train your mind, and to discover things about yourself and the world.

Meditation as a Means of Feeling Better

The main reason people come to meditation is that they want to feel better in some way. Everyone likes to feel better, and meditation works. Many people have heard about or seen the evidence that meditation can be good for relaxation and stress relief. It is. But there are many other ways it improves your wellbeing beyond relaxation and stress relief.

I started meditating regularly during a difficult time at university. I was in my second year at Cambridge and had started having panic attacks. A friend suggested I try meditating. I wasn't new to meditation, but I didn't have a regular practice. He had taken some courses with one of the big meditation organizations, Transcendental Meditation® (often referred to as TM), liked it, and recommended I try it. I learned the TM method, started practicing, and it worked. I started feeling noticeably better within a week, and the panic attacks stopped. I'm not trying to prescribe meditation for panic attacks, but it worked for me.

Most people that come to my classes aren't suffering from something as acute as panic attacks, but many feel overwhelmed, out of control, stressed, or anxious. Others are trying meditation because they have heard it makes people happier.

Regardless of why people come to my meditation classes, most of them say they enjoy it. They say it makes them feel more relaxed and at peace. They say it gives them more clarity, a sense of spaciousness in their mind, and better emotional balance. For many, this experience is good enough for them to come back to another class, or to start their own daily practice at home.

Just the act of sitting still and breathing properly triggers a relaxation response in your body. The exercises involved in meditation build on that. Over the long-term, these changes can be profound. People's daily baseline of happiness ends up much higher.

Meditation can't eliminate the hardships of life. They happen to everyone. Meditation can help you deal with the hardships better, and to recover faster when you get knocked down. It also helps you get more enjoyment out of the good parts of life.

Meditation as a Training

All the meditation techniques I've tried will make you feel better. Some meditation techniques also work as a training.

Most people agree that some sort of exercise is important for your physical health. Meditation is an equivalent training for your mental health. Different types of physical training develop different aspects of your fitness like endurance, strength, or flexibility. Different meditation techniques develop different aspects of your mental and emotional fitness with benefits across every aspect of your life.

There are two principle things that are trained through meditation: your *awareness* and your *compassion*.

Training Your Awareness

As you are reading this book, there are a number of things you may be aware of. You may be aware of the sounds around you. You may be aware of whether you are hungry, or thirsty. You may be aware of your feelings about this book.

In class, I like to try to introduce the concept of awareness, as distinct from thinking, by asking people to listen to some music. When you hear a song, if you pay close attention to the sound, listening carefully to the notes, the flow, the melodies, and allow the music to wash over you, *without* thinking about it, you are aware of the music. If you start to analyze the music, if you wonder what key it's in or try to identify which instruments are being used, you are no longer in that state of awareness of the music, now you are thinking about it.

Sometimes a beautiful sunset, a view from the top of a mountain, or sitting beside the ocean can cause us to pause. We have a moment where we aren't thinking about what we're seeing and experiencing, we are just observing the scene, without thinking. That is awareness. Our attention is fully in the moment, observing what is present right now.

Then, we might start to think about what we are observing. We might compare it to other beautiful things we've seen, or start to think about who we wish were sharing this moment with us. Maybe we want to try to capture the moment; we take a picture, share it over the Internet, and hope that people can enjoy it with us. This is thinking. We have gone from a direct experience of the world outside us to an experience that is in our head where we are thinking about the world outside us.

Meditation helps us distinguish between these states of consciousness. One involves our open awareness of what is going on right now. The other involves thinking, evaluating, worrying, and considering.

Thinking, evaluating, worrying, and considering are important things for us to be able to do. They help us survive, have friends, do our jobs, and define who we are as people. We may think of these as being our conscious activities, but ironically these conscious activities happen unconsciously. By that, I mean that our thoughts tend to happen automatically whether we want them to or not. This is what the story of the man on the horse is about. We are not directing our thinking, our worrying, our evaluations, or our considerations. They happen, and we are along for the ride.

Many meditation techniques are really just different ways of helping us to start to notice when we are thinking. Some meditation techniques are also good at helping us become more familiar with present moment awareness.

You may think, "of course I'm aware of things," and you are, but in awareness training, you are going to expand your understanding of what that means, and what your 'awareness' can include.

Awareness Training Part One: *The Breath*

Awareness training traditionally starts with breathing. It is a simple and yet powerful technique. You start with trying to hold your attention on the act of breathing in, and out. Almost immediately your mind will get distracted and start thinking about something else. Then, at some point, you will become aware that you are no longer focused on the breathing.

Awareness Training Part Two: *Thoughts*

The moment you are aware you are no longer focused on the breathing is a critical moment in meditation. It is a brief moment of awareness, awareness of your own mind and its thoughts.

Most of the time we aren't aware of our thoughts. Most of the time we are carried away with our thoughts. We like them, we agree with everything they say. We allow them to run wherever they want, assuming that they are who we are. Yet in the moment when you are aware of your attention having gone somewhere other than where you have put it, you touch into your *observing mind* that sits slightly separate from the thoughts themselves. This is the moment when you start to become aware that you and your thoughts may have a very close relationship, but they are not exactly the same thing. You have the ability to be aware of your own thoughts, and that awareness is independent of the thinking mind itself.

Awareness Training Part Three: *The Body*

Another meditation that helps to develop awareness is to bring the attention to the physical sensations of the body.

With the possible exception of athletes and dancers, most of us live our lives 'in our heads,' right behind our eyes. We have a body, but we are not particularly aware of it except when it forces us to notice it. If we are hungry, tired, or in pain then we pay attention, but other than that we are unaware of it.

This next step of awareness training helps us to become more aware of our bodies on a moment-to-moment basis. There are specific meditation techniques where we scan the body and notice what it is sensing. Once we tune in and pay attention, we notice it is continually sensing a lot more than we realize. Almost every part of your body is sending you information, but it isn't terribly 'important' information, so we ignore it. One of the useful aspects of body scan meditation is that the information the body is sending is always real-time information. Unlike our thoughts which are often thinking about the past, or worrying about the future, our body is only giving us sensations right now. As we click in to pay attention, we are automatically moving more into a state of awareness and doing less thinking.

Awareness Training Part Four: *Emotions*

Different from the physical sensations of your body are the emotions you are feeling. Again, like our awareness of our bodies, many of us are not particularly aware of our emotions at any particular moment. We feel our emotions are annoyances that interfere with our logical, rational approach to life. Emotions are to be overcome or to be ignored. Yet when you pause during meditation and notice what feelings and emotions are present, whether they be anxiety, excitement, sadness, anger, jealousy, happiness, or joy, or even a complex combination of many of them at the same time, you can start to give them space, learn more about them, to manage your reactions to them, and even to use them.

Awareness Training Part Five: *Stimulus and Response*

A common scenario: You sit down to meditate. You're trying to hold attention on the breath. You lose it and follow a thought for a while before realizing you are thinking. You bring your attention back to the breath. This goes on for a few minutes. Then your phone vibrates.

In awareness training, the instruction right then would be to see if you can notice your reaction to the phone. Can you notice the feeling arising from within? You probably want to check it, to see what the message is. You might feel an urgency. You might feel anxiety, anticipation, or excitement that it could be important.

There is nothing wrong with checking the phone of course, but what is interesting from a training perspective is to become aware of that reaction as it appears. Something happened – the phone beeped with an alert – and then something else happened in response – the urge to check it.

It doesn't have to be a phone. Any meditation session of more than a couple of minutes is going to have different things happen. You may develop an itch. You may get bored, or frustrated. You may suddenly feel you have too much to do today, and you need to finish the meditation early to get on with it. All these are common experiences during meditation.

In the beginning, we don't necessarily see these feelings as they arise, but we can notice them once they have come. We can start to develop the awareness of what has changed within us; that we now feel the powerful desire to scratch, to move, or to stop meditating.

Throughout our day, throughout our lives, things are constantly happening that cause reactions in us. We go past a bakery, and the smell triggers a sense of hunger or a craving for that taste of fresh, warm bread. A driver in front of us does something stupid, and anger arises. A colleague says something dismissive, and we feel insulted, sad, or fearful. Our reactions may be normal and well justified, but meditation helps us develop our awareness of these reactions as they occur.

Viktor Frankl was a psychiatrist who wrote inspirationally about what he learned from his horrific experiences in concentration camps like Auschwitz. One of his more famous quotes about human potential is:

> *"Between stimulus and response there is a space.*
> *In that space is our power to choose our response.*
> *In our response lies our growth and our freedom."*

Meditation, and specifically the training of our awareness of our reactions to changes, helps us to find that critical space between stimulus and response.

Training Your Compassion

I am always nervous before I introduce the second main aspect that meditation trains, that of compassion. I get nervous because the word compassion can have moral overtones. I have no agenda in trying to change who you are or trying to encourage you to become a nicer, more generous, or softer person. Compassion training can change you, but any change will be your choice, and training in compassion is not going to do anything except what you allow it to do. Yet it can be powerful and profound, with more benefits than you expect.

The starting supposition of this training is that you are not so much developing compassion, as you are uncovering your innate capacity for it. You were born with this capacity for compassion, but perhaps you don't practice it as much as you might. In certain meditations, often referred to as loving kindness meditations, we bring it forward and give it a workout.

In my classes, compassion training follows awareness training because there is something I want people to be able to notice. I start by inviting people to bring someone to mind that they care about unconditionally. Then I invite them to send them loving thoughts and feelings (there's a technique for this that we'll look at later). After a few minutes of this, I then ask them to direct that same love and compassion toward themselves.

The moment I ask people to send themselves love and compassion is always tricky. I look forward to it and dread it in almost equal amounts. I look forward to it because it is a powerful moment of realization for people, but I dread it because the mood of the room changes instantly. It is almost as though someone has dropped a glass on the floor and it shatters. Everyone stops for a second. There is a palpable resistance in the room to what I have asked them to do. This is where the awareness training kicks in as I encourage people to notice how resistant they are to giving themselves that same degree of compassion they would freely give to someone they care about.

Most of us are very conscious of our failings and imperfections, and we feel unworthy of that level of love. For some, there is resistance because it feels self-indulgent to give ourselves that love or there is a sense of guilt associated with giving that generosity to oneself instead of to someone else. I encourage people to be aware of the resistance, and to notice it but ask them to try to avoid thinking about the resistance, or where it might have come from. Then I ask them to see if they can relax that resistance for a few minutes and send themselves love and compassion anyway. There is more to the compassion training than this, but in my introductory classes, the big emphasis is on helping people lower their resistance to this self-compassion.

The effect of this is profound. Consider how many of the nasty things people do to each other, as well as the incredibly destructive things we do to ourselves, that might be prevented if everyone felt a little better about themselves. It won't solve all the world's problems, but it could prevent, or heal, a great deal of suffering. You might think this is as simple as saying "everyone should be nicer to themselves," but it turns out this is not easy. In fact, it is very hard for most people. It takes training to learn how to do this. Compassion training using loving kindness meditation offers that training. And there is a lot more available from compassion training than just feeling better about yourself as we'll see later.

Focus, Curiosity, and Non-Judgment

In addition to awareness and compassion, there are three attributes to develop that help us meditate, and also help us in our daily lives. Our focus, curiosity, and non-judgment.

Focus

Focus is the continued holding of attention on a single thing. When we meditate, our focus is being worked continuously. In a breath meditation, we start by trying to hold our attention on the breathing. The mind gets distracted and wanders off. At some point, we notice that our focus is no longer on the breath. When we notice we are no longer focused on our breathing, we gently return our focus back to the next breath.

Three things are getting trained here; initially we are training our minds to hold focus, then we are training it to notice when we have lost focus, and finally, we are developing the skill of moving our focus back to where we want it to be. Becoming more aware of where our focus is from moment-to-moment, and developing that skill of moving it where we want can change many aspects of our daily lives.

Curiosity

If I were asked what I know now that I wish I'd known at the beginning of my meditation career, it would be the value of curiosity. Looking back, I can see there were many times I was told to encourage and utilize curiosity, but I didn't hear it in quite those terms until relatively recently.

A few years ago, I found myself at a nine-day Mindfulness Based Stress Reduction (MBSR) seminar. MBSR is a program set up by Jon Kabat-Zinn in the 1970s and is now one of largest programs that teach meditation outside of a religious context. The explosion of interest in meditation as a secular activity is largely thanks to MBSR, and I love what they have done and continue to do. However, at this event, some things had gone wrong. I was disappointed that it seemed to have been a waste of time, and I was feeling very critical of the event. At some point during the seminar, we spent two days in complete silence which seemed only to help ripen my self-righteousness and develop it into full-fledged anger against them for ruining the seminar and against myself for making the mistake of coming. With no TV, no internet, no email, no phone, and no distractions of any kind my anger bubbled away, getting stronger and stronger.

One of the facilitators of the retreat was Judson Brewer, who is one of the preeminent neuroscientists looking into meditation. He was giving guidance before one of the meditation sessions and encouraged us to use curiosity as a way of dealing with pain, or as a way of sitting with unpleasant emotions. He pointed out that when we feel uncomfortable the usual responses for most humans are to suppress the feeling, to distract ourselves, or to try to change the feeling by doing something like eating, drinking, watching TV, calling a friend, or whatever. Instead, he encouraged us to do what seemed like the opposite. He suggested that instead of turning away from it, ignoring it, or trying to suppress it, we could try looking at it more closely, exploring the feeling in detail, and to use that childlike quality of curiosity to investigate it.

I had nothing to lose except my rage, so I gave it a go. It took a while since it was a new approach for me at the time, but slowly as I moved into the anger inside my mind and body, it started to unravel. It still had a great charge on it, but it lost some of its hold on my state of mind. I started to be able to separate the angry thoughts from the angry feelings. I didn't like the anger and was resisting it as well as reacting to it with my mind, but as my thoughts separated slightly from the feeling I started to be able to feel the anger, and to become aware of it simply as it was, a feeling. A very uncomfortable feeling to be sure, but I started to see and experience it just as the energy that it was and let it flow throughout my body without suppressing it. It felt very hot. I still didn't like it, but as I let it flow I could feel its power. I noticed a surprising sense of awe in me in recognition of the energy it held. I also noticed that as it flowed, it started to lose its power, eventually burning itself out, and the feeling went away.

What now seems obvious to me about this is that when we feel joy, we let it flow through us. There is no suppression or running away from it; we let it be. We enjoy it. And then what happens? It goes away. As I've learned, whatever uncomfortable feelings I might be feeling, if I approach them with curiosity, and then let them flow through me, they also go away. It doesn't mean I like them. When I wake up in a bad mood, I still feel a resistance and resentment towards whatever I'm feeling. I also don't like the concept of 'accepting' them, but have learned, thanks to Judson, to 'acknowledge' them, to approach them, get curious about them, sit with them, and eventually they change and go away.

Curiosity is more than simply a way to deal with difficult emotions, but that is how I first came to appreciate it. It is also a useful technique for improving focus and awareness during meditation. It also has many benefits for our real life.

Non-Judgment

Non-judgment is tricky. For a start, it's *not doing* something. It's also not doing something that we are programmed to do. All day we are using our judgment to decide what we like or dislike, agree with or disagree with, what we need to have and what we need to avoid. Non-judgment is the practice of not doing any of those things. There are a number of reasons it is valuable to develop this through meditation.

One characteristic of our judgment is that it tends to happen automatically. Something happens, and we judge it, almost immediately. There is nothing wrong with judgment, per se; it is a critical component of who we are and of our survival. But what we try to develop in meditation is the ability to turn that automatic reaction into a conscious activity. An activity that we can use when we want, and one we can suspend when we want.

Non-judgment is a helpful skill to develop for our lives but it is also an important component for developing our meditation practice. As we try to develop our awareness, which is about being focused only on what is present right now and aware of what is arising in each moment, you need to be able to put judgment on hold. It is easier said than done. Nevertheless, it is important to try to observe your mind, your body, your emotions, your breath, your thoughts with as little judgment as possible. For one thing, the aspect of mind which does the thinking is by being engaged the moment you judge anything, and the simple awareness is gone. Training ourselves in non-judgment is a way of helping to notice, and prevent some of the mind's activity during our practice.

Meditation as Discovery

There isn't as much to say here except there is another dimension to meditation other than feeling better and the training aspects. Feeling better, and training can be attractive to people. Yet as people start meditation practice I ask them to be open to the possibility that they will discover, or perhaps uncover, many other things that weren't mentioned.

Some meditation techniques involve turning inward and you will learn more about yourself. As you become more aware of your thoughts, your impulses, and your reactions you will start to see patterns. You will learn more about what makes you tick, and about what ticks you off.

Some of these discoveries are sufficiently universal that I can point them out, like learning to see your own thoughts. However, one of the most exciting things about meditation is that over time you will discover many other things on your own, and those discoveries may be unique to you.

When in Burgundy, Florian our guide pointed out all sorts of things that we might not have noticed, but there was a lot he did not point out. Like Florian, I am pointing out certain things that I find interesting, or that I have found useful, but I'm not showing you all of what meditation offers. There is a lot more to uncover that is for you to find out. Everyone is different, and I cannot predict what you will find except that I urge you to be open to what happens.

For some people, meditation leads them to a better sense of who they are, deep down. To the extent that people may not feel entirely fulfilled, it could be because they are not living their lives in accordance with their deeper values and passions.

When we meditate we quiet some of the outside voices and external influences that can confuse us as to who we are, what we should be doing, or how we should be living. What is left is our own truth. These discoveries often happen gradually and don't necessarily result in drastic upheaval.

It isn't so much that people quit their jobs and join the Peace Corps, but it might be that they finally make the time to exercise, take a guitar lesson, or make more effort with their families; or even that that they find themselves more focused, in a new way, on their work as they rediscover their passion for what they do.

Having suggested that one of the discoveries you might make could be related to your deeper self, I don't want to limit it to that either. There could be any number of discoveries so long as you remain open to more than what you think is on offer. Most of the world's religions have contemplative practices, including meditation, within their traditions. Some see these contemplative practices as leading to an experience of something other, which they might talk about as God. Others refer to experiences of transcendence and of the mystical unity of all of reality.

What is consistent across the different traditions, throughout history, is that people have had experiences from which they have drawn enormous conclusions as to the nature of the universe and the purpose of life. It is not the objective of this book to draw any such conclusions, but I hope that you might stay open to the possibility that meditation has more to offer than just feeling better, or even just as a training. Those are worthwhile reasons to meditate, but there may be other experiences, insights, or wisdom to be discovered.

CHAPTER TWO

Relationships
PART ONE: Making Connection

Memory is peculiar. I can't remember someone's name as soon as they've told me, but there are events from years ago where I still recall every detail. Meeting a certain girl in the fall of 1989 was one of those moments.

It was a crisp but sunny morning. She was standing on the other side of the road from me, near the Senate House in Cambridge, England. I had heard a great deal about her in the few weeks since term had started. It seemed like every guy that met her had fallen in love. They would gush about how incredible she was, how charming, intelligent, and beautiful. She had been pointed out to me at a distance, but I hadn't had the chance to meet her until now. She was talking to a friend of mine, and I decided to introduce myself.

I was nervous because part of me didn't want to fall under the same spell as everyone else, yet part of me did – who doesn't like falling in love? I was surprised because as I got closer, I wasn't sure what the excitement was about. I'd assumed she would be some kind of supermodel. She was pretty, but far more normal looking than I'd expected.

I crossed the street and approached on the pretense of saying hello to my friend. He sighed as I approached, which I read as his disappointment at my interruption, but he introduced us. I tried to be as casual as possible and pretend I didn't know who she was, and we all exchanged pleasantries for a few minutes. Then I found myself walking away in a daze, almost stumbling, shocked and confused as to what had just happened. She hadn't flirted, and she hadn't been particularly funny. Nothing profound had been discussed, it was merely the normal chit chat about which college you were in, what you were studying, etc., but it had happened. I was in love. What was the secret of this woman that made me and everyone else fall for her as soon as they met her?

A few years ago, I found myself on a meditation retreat where I had a similar experience. It was near the end of the retreat, after several days of silence, and we were doing an exercise to ease us back into the real world.

The facilitator asked us to consider a few questions such as how the retreat had affected us, what we'd liked, and whether we were excited or nervous about returning to our regular lives. We were then invited to turn to someone near us and to share our answers but in a very specific way. The instruction was for one person to talk for three minutes. The person listening was to sit in silence, not interrupting, not asking clarifying questions, not adding to what they had said, not agreeing with them or even reacting with a nod or a smile. We were not to participate in the conversation in any way except to listen. An extra part of the instruction was that the listener had to pay attention very closely because at the end of the three minutes they were going to try to repeat back what the first person had said, as close to word for word as they could. When the listener was repeating back what they'd heard there was to be no interpretation, no guessing as to what the first person had meant. We had to try to remember the actual words used. The advice was to try to listen without mentally interpreting what the other person was saying. Simply listen to the words.

I paired up with the woman sitting next to me, and we started. She went first, and I listened. I repeated back to her what she'd said, using as many of the words, terms, and phrases as I could remember. She clarified a couple of things I had got wrong, and then it was my turn. I spoke, she listened and then she repeated back to me as closely as she could what she'd heard. As she repeated back what I'd said, I noticed intense feelings of connection, energy, intimacy, attraction, and even love pouring through me. I didn't know her. I couldn't particularly 'like' her. I certainly couldn't be 'falling in love' with her, and yet it was the same feeling as I'd had on that street corner all those years before while I was at university. After the listening exercise, many people commented in surprise that they had had similar experiences while their partners were repeating back what they had said.

We Love it When People Listen

It turns out that having someone listen to you is both surprisingly powerful, and incredibly rare. When I ask my meditation class to think of people they know who are really good listeners, most can only think of one or two people. I then ask them to consider what they think about these people and the response is overwhelmingly positive. We value people who listen, in part because they are so unusual.

As human beings, we are social creatures, and we like making connections with others. We want to experience intimacy and have close friends. We want people to think well of us. We often go about this by talking, by having people listen to what we say, trying to impress them with our intelligence, our wit, our insights, or because of our importance, our friends, and our exciting social life. One problem is that everyone is trying to do the same. Everyone in our society seems to be constantly talking, sharing relentlessly about every aspect of their life.

What made the girl at university special was that she wasn't trying to impress you with what she had to say. She impressed by having an ability to listen to what you were saying as though it mattered to her. She was listening without agenda. She wasn't waiting patiently for you to stop talking so that she could talk. She wasn't being polite. She was genuinely interested in what you had to say. She made everyone feel valuable, as though they mattered, that they had been seen, heard and appreciated. It was so unusual and so powerful that everyone fell in love with her.

When you first start dating someone and fall in love, it is a wonderful period of discovery. You meet someone who shares certain values and interests and who you find interesting enough to really listen to. If you are lucky they are also interested in you, they will ask you questions about yourself and then listen to the answers. On one level intimacy is as simple as that. People talking, and listening. Of course, there are complexities of attraction, pheromones, etc., but the power of intimacy is defined by the power of the listening. Then, sadly, at some point in the development of a relationship, the magical spark of falling in love fades. So does your interest in every word they have to say, as does theirs in what you have to say.

It may be tempting to think that the intensity with which we listen is the result of how passionately we still feel about the other person. However, the relationship between our listening and how we feel is not one way. We fall in love partly because we are being heard, and we fall out of love when we stop being heard. A large part of couples' therapy is simply about getting people to start listening to each other again.

If you are lucky, you have a few close friends. What defines those friendships may appear to be your common history, interests or activities. Perhaps you went to school together, you work together, go to the gym together, shop together, or that you both share the same political beliefs, have kids the same age, or are both single. Commonalities like these can forge the initial connections, but real friendships are formed when people listen to each other. We may think that our friends listen to us because they are our friends, but really they are our friends because they listen to us.

Good listening is so rare that many of us have to pay money to get it in the form of counselors, coaches, or therapists. There is a lot more to therapy than listening of course, but a critical part of a therapist's training is learning to listen. Their goal is to develop a close relationship that allows trust, honesty, and vulnerability to arise so that healing can begin. This relationship is developed through listening and having the client feel he or she is being heard.

If we don't see therapists, we might go to a bar, where the bar person and the people sitting beside us have agreed via some cultural norm that they will let us talk. They haven't been trained to listen, and they don't really care, but they let us talk and pretend to appear vaguely interested.

We all want to talk and to be heard by other people, yet we have to make do with the talking part. Good listening is hard to come by which is strange since we can all do it.

We Aren't Good at Listening;
We Aren't Even Good at Fake Listening

I used to teach people about the importance of listening when I worked as a corporate trainer. I would start by breaking the class into small groups to discuss whether they could tell whether someone wasn't listening to them. Everyone would agree they know when someone is not listening. Then I would ask how they know. There are certain easy giveaways such as someone looking at their phone (or even typing away) while you're talking. Sometimes they are repeatedly glancing over your shoulder to see if there is someone else more important to talk to. It may be that their body language is closed.

After the group had explored the obvious ways, I would ask them if they had had the experience of someone doing all the things a person is supposed to do while listening such as looking you in the eye, with open body language, occasionally nodding or murmuring agreement and yet you still know they aren't really listening. Everyone again would agree that they could tell when someone is not really listening, even if the listener is doing all the right things. Then the key question was whether they thought people could tell when they weren't listening. I would pause to let the point sink in, and soon there would be nervous giggling as everyone realized they probably haven't been fooling anyone.

We often think we are being polite and clever when we fake listen, but if the other person is vaguely aware and paying attention, then they will know. It's rare that someone will call you on it, but that doesn't mean you've fooled anyone. Most people are good at telling when people aren't really listening, and the flip side is that we probably aren't as good at fake listening as we think we are.

The training exercise I used to do wasn't wrong per se, but it assumed that listening is in our control. In the exercise, I was pointing out to people that if they want to appear as though they are listening, they actually have to be listening. The implication was that people have the ability to listen provided they decide to make the effort. However, unless we've been trained, the chances are that we are not as good at listening as we think we are, even if we are trying. Listening is much harder than most people realize. This is where meditation comes in. Meditation can show you how bad you are at listening, and it shows you why you are bad at listening. It can train you to be better.

Listening is Hard

When you meditate for the first time, you discover that your mind is not under your control as much as you might have thought. You sit down and try to focus on something like your breathing, or on a phrase that you repeat over and over. Yet your mind wanders off almost immediately and seemingly of its own accord. In meditation, there is the instruction to try to notice when this has happened and to bring your attention back to the point of focus, over and over again, every time it happens. If you catch yourself quickly enough, this can happen twenty or thirty times in a ten-minute session. Exactly the same thing is happening when you are listening to someone except it is even worse. You might be trying to stay focused on what they are saying, but your mind wants to jump in different directions. In meditation, the distractions are only in your mind and yet it is hard to stay focused. When someone is talking they are continually giving you extra things to think about, to consider, to evaluate, to judge, and to decide if you agree, disagree, like, or dislike. The moment your mind goes down one of those tracks, you are no longer paying attention to what they are saying. If we disagree with what they are saying, we stop listening to what they are now talking about and start formulating what we are going to say when they stop. Or perhaps they say something that reminds us of something completely different, like we need to call someone back, or remember to pick up dog food on the way home. This is all happening on the occasions when we are genuinely trying to listen.

Much of the time we don't really want to listen. We want to talk and be listened to. Therefore, we might hear something the other person is saying and start thinking about what we can talk about which is far more interesting than what this person is saying. Then we look for the moment when we can cut in. Alternatively, we may decide that we know what they are saying and we don't need to listen. It would be rude at this point to tell them to shut up because they're boring, so we switch off and think about something completely different.

Recently I was going to teach meditation at a local church. The church was hosting a number of community activities that evening, meditation being one, and they served a light dinner for everyone beforehand. I sat down at a table, and a conversation started about where people were from and how they'd ended up attending this particular church. A woman explained she'd been raised Presbyterian but ended up Episcopal. A man then said he'd had a similar history. There was a follow-up question asking what that history was. His answer started innocently enough by saying that he used to go to a Greek Orthodox Church. Without any follow-up questions, or even much of a pause, he was still talking many minutes later (though it felt like hours). We had received a detailed analysis of the reasons why he had left the Orthodox Church. He had explained about some of the dogmatic differences between Russian and Greek Orthodox churches. We had 'heard' about what the priests were like, and the love-hate relationship this person maintained with his old church.

I expect (and hope) not everyone around the table was as critical as I was. I think I was particularly judgmental because I do exactly the same thing where I can take an innocent, polite, chit chat question and launch myself into an exposition, fascinated by my own opinions. However, my point of this story is to reveal what was going through my head as he was talking, because I wasn't listening. I heard the words, and I can remember the essence of what he was talking about, but inside my head was a much louder conversation.

"Wow, that's kind of interesting." I thought when he started. Yet my brain almost immediately started to see how I could orient what he was saying towards me.

"I've been to a Greek Orthodox service. It was pretty cool. All the smells, the smoke, the candles. I should let them know I've done that. I wonder how I can weave my story into his when he stops for a minute. I could show how smart I am, show that the meditation guy knows about Greek Orthodoxy. I don't, but I could look as though I do. I could talk about the iconography and its similarity to Tibetan Buddhist pictures of saints. That would sound intelligent. Maybe pretentious. No, I'm sure it would look clever. Maybe this would steer the conversation towards meditation."

After not very much longer my judging self kicked in,

"Wow, he's really going on. Now he's off talking about the Russian church. Does he really think we are interested?"

"Jeez, when is he going to stop? Has he taken a breath? How can he keep going like this?"

"I need to go soon, how can I politely get out of this? Is that a pause? Can I go now? No."

"OH MY GOD, he's still talking! What planet is he on that he thinks he has the right to dominate a conversation like this?"

"Maybe I could include this in the chapter on communication somehow."

My point is not that he was a bad guy for talking the way he did, nor particularly to reveal what a jerk I am inside my head. It is that when we think we are listening, our mind is going all over the place, in the same way as it goes all over the place when we are meditating. When you are meditating there is no extra stimulus for your mind to run off in different directions, but it does anyway. When you are listening, you have your usual, highly distractible mind, plus all the stuff they are saying to you as extra objects for your thoughts to run with, or to judge. It's as though we are listening to them with headphones on, the headphones being much louder and playing the thoughts of our own mind. We can still get the gist of what they are saying, but it isn't coming through clearly, and we are more interested in our words than we are in theirs. Sometimes we might decide not to listen, but most of the time we're not deciding not to listen, we're just not listening.

Listening is harder than we think it is. The mind is good at processing, thinking, judging, analyzing, redirecting our attention to wherever it wants to go. We think we're very clever; we can do all that processing, thinking, judging, analyzing, anticipating, and redirecting at the same time as we are listening. And we can ... to an extent, but we are fooling ourselves if we think we are really listening while that is going on. We're partially listening. In order to really listen, you have to stay present with what they're saying in each moment. This goes against the natural inclination of the mind. Even if you want to listen, it is hard if not impossible without training. You need a training that helps you become aware of your mind's wandering; you need training in bringing your mind's focus back where you want it to be, in this case on the listening. Meditation is that training.

Just because you meditate doesn't mean you will suddenly become a perfect listener. I meditate, and I don't listen all the time. I still get distracted; I get bored, I judge, I get frustrated that a conversation isn't all about me. What meditation has given me is the ability to click in and listen a lot better when I want to. I still get distracted while I'm listening, but because of meditation training I become aware of those distractions and can redirect my focus back to what is currently being said. It isn't easy, but it is possible.

Back at the end of the meditation retreat when we did the listening exercise, and everyone fell in love, we had been meditating several hours a day for many days. On retreat, you have no distractions to get you out of your head. You become hyper aware of your thoughts, their patterns and the paths they go down. You also get less attached to these thoughts. With nothing else to distract your attention, you start to notice that most of your thoughts are the same and are like songs on endless repeat cycles that you keep playing over and over. After a while with nothing else to listen to, your thoughts become less interesting, even boring, so that you start to let go of them and find the peace and calm on the other side of the relentless chatter in your head. So by the time we did the exercise we were primed to be far more present to the person in front of us, rather than interrupting them in our heads with our own conversation. There were some other helpful pointers.

One was to avoid judgment of what the person is saying while they are saying it. This is easier said than done since our minds love judging and usually do it automatically. Learning how to notice our judgments, how to let go of them, and even avoid them in the first place is another key part of meditation training. In true listening, we try to put our judgment on hold. Only once we have fully heard the person do we then evaluate, but it is critical to separate the two activities.

Another helpful guideline we received was to try to avoid 'interpreting' what the person was saying while they were saying it. Interpretation requires evaluation, consideration, and judgment. Instead, we were invited to simply listen to the words and to see if we could repeat back as closely as possible the exact words we heard. When you are really trying to listen, this is a useful trick. Focus merely on what is being said by the other person, the exact words, rather than what is going on in your head.

The final aspect of meditation training that is useful is to approach the listening with curiosity. Curiosity can help put our evaluating, thinking, wandering mind on hold as we use curiosity to really get close and observe what they are saying, and how they are saying it in as detailed a way as we can, without judging. If you approach the listening as though you were going to have to describe it in as much detail as possible, not only the exact words but the body language, the tone, pace, and volume of the language you will find yourself paying attention more closely.

Focus, noticing when our mind is distracted, refocusing the mind, using curiosity and avoiding judgment. If you want to be the rare exception of the person who can listen, these are the skills to develop. These are the skills you develop in meditation.

You Can't Always Get What You Want, but if You Try Sometimes ...

I play golf. One aspect of the game is that you are stuck with someone's company for several hours as you go around the course. It can be an opportunity to deepen a friendship with someone you already know, but I also like to show up on my own sometimes and get paired with someone I don't know. I like that it gives me an opportunity to test my listening skills and see if I can pay attention to what they are saying. I challenge myself to see how much I can remember of what they've said at the end of the round. Creating that challenge for myself helps me to focus my listening and allows us to form a real connection. However, there are occasions where I will have asked many questions and listened to what they have to say. I will know a lot about them, but at the end of the round, they won't know a single thing about me, having not asked even one question.

The truth for most of us is that we want to be listened to, we don't really want to be the one doing the listening. This is part of the reason there is not much listening going on. Learning to listen and becoming one of the few people that are really paying attention while someone is talking is not necessarily what you want. You want them to listen to you.

This gives you a choice. You can continue to talk at people, pretending to yourself that they are listening. Or you can start to be one of the few that are making real connections by being a person that listens. That gets you half way towards really meeting people mentally and emotionally.

You and I may never get good enough at this that everyone falls in love when they talk to us, but it nevertheless has the power to change every relationship in your life.

Your friendships can start to develop and go to new levels. Your friends feel the same as you do, they want to be heard, seen, listened to, and appreciated. You are going to develop the skill to make that happen.

If you are in a relationship, you are going to be able to rekindle the intimacy that has dissipated over time.

If you are single but looking for love, your dates will suddenly find you far more interesting and attractive. Not because you're more interesting and attractive but because they will feel more interesting and attractive in your company since you genuinely listened to them.

Listening is one of the greatest gifts you can give another person. You are giving them the sense that they matter. It is as simple as listening, once you realize that listening is not easy. It can be learned; however, it is not something you can do just because you choose to. Your mind wanders too much. Train your mind to focus, to pay attention, to notice when it is wandering and then to refocus. Meditate, and you can become a better listener.

CHAPTER THREE

Relationships
PART TWO: Managing Conflict

It's a Saturday evening and I'm feeling stressed. Work is not going well and every project is behind schedule, including this book which was supposed to be finished by now. I had hoped to have corporate clients for my training business by now. Hackers have somehow started registering on my website even while it languishes "Under Construction" and there isn't even a page to register on. My hopes and expectations for where I should be are entirely of my own creation and yet I feel like I am failing. I picture friends and family being disapproving about how little I've accomplished. Even though this disapproval only exists in my brain, I am deeply resentful of it. It is also 'date night' with my girlfriend, which is not going well.

Sally and I like to cook, or at least I think we do. It's not that we're great at it, but it's an activity we do together, a little bonding exercise where we end up creating something, and then we get to sit down and enjoy it. It's my favorite type of date night and tonight is my attempt to reconnect our relationship after a week where we've been too busy to catch up.

I say I like cooking, and I do most of the time, but sometimes it causes me stress. I'm a relatively new cook, so I don't have complete confidence that things will turn out okay and I struggle with the timing. Ideally, everything is ready at exactly the same time, but if you start the broccoli too early it either over cooks or goes cold. If you start the spuds too late, then everything has to wait, or you have lumpy, raw, mashed potatoes.

Tonight, we're taking a bit of a risk and trying a recipe we haven't done before, so I'm already nervous and have no idea how the timings need to go. I've planned it out, but we've started later than I'd expected (because I was trying to fix all my other projects) and I feel like we need to catch up. Instead of being all nice, sweet, kind, and romantic I'm starting to get terse, bossy, and short tempered. Sally is far more easy going (which is rubbing me the wrong way right now) and is casually reading the recipe. "We don't have time for that." I think, for no good reason except that I am feeling like we are going to end up eating later than I'd planned, later than we should, and later than the imaginary people in my head would find acceptable.

"Why don't you do the carrots and parsnips?" I say, getting them out and dropping them on the counter for her.

"Okay." She says.

I sense that she is probably aware I'm not in the best of moods. I feel bad about that since tonight is supposed to be all about us, but hope she hasn't really noticed. I get on with the garlic and onions.

As is inevitable when trying to rush, it's one of those days when whatever you try to do quickly goes slowly. I am trying to peel, slice, and crush the garlic as fast as possible, but it is very fresh, so the bulbs are sticking to their skins and refusing to come out. My frustration builds. Eventually, I have the garlic and onions ready and turn to check on Sally. The recipe has called for the parsnips and carrots to be cut into large pieces that will be roasted. Sally has diced them into small pieces.

"What the f?" I think. "Didn't you read the f'ing recipe?"

I think I'm being noble by keeping my thoughts to myself. Instead, I sigh. One of those "I'm really disappointed in you" sort of sighs.

"Err, they weren't supposed to be diced. But I'm sure it'll be okay." I am looking down at the floor. If I were a cartoon right now, steam would be coming out of my ears. I am trying not to get angry, but instead of allowing the evening to develop however it develops, I start acting all superior. I make it clear that when this meal doesn't work, it won't have been my fault. It will have been her fault. As a master of the passive aggressive communication style, I can convey all this without words. I move around too fast, bumping into her often and carelessly, and make lots of noise as I drop saucepans and trays down harder than I need to. I go out to start the barbecue, which I realize is now going to be ready far too late for everything else. I'm furious for no good reason at all. Sally is upset because she thinks I'm upset with her. Date night is all but ruined. The food, of course, turned out just fine.

Even with the best of intentions relationships can be difficult. This is a trivial example of how conflict can erupt between two people that do still love each other, but even as it was happening, there was a part of me watching the drama unfold. It sat back, amused that someone writing a book about meditation could completely botch a romantic moment as thoroughly as I was doing. There are much harder obstacles for relationships to navigate such as finances, religion, children, illness, or looking after parents. Smaller but highly animated disagreements can be about where to live, where to go on holiday, décor, socks on the floor, dishes in the sink, taking out the garbage, toilet seats up or down, who does the laundry, or who gets to hold the remote control. We are social creatures that want companionship, but companionship comes with conflict. Meditation is a helpful way to get closer and more intimate with people by teaching you how to be more present, to listen better, to be more sensitive to the person in front of you, but it doesn't mean everything is going to go smoothly. Nevertheless, when it comes to conflict (and despite my apparent incompetence), meditation does help. It can't always prevent conflicts from happening, but it can make them happen less often, be less damaging when they occur, and help you recover more quickly. To see how, let's have a quick look at some of the reasons why conflict is inevitable in the first place.

The 2-Year Old Architect of Your Psyche

From the moment we are born, we are trying to make sense of the world, and we are discovering ways to get our needs met. At first, this might be as basic as crying whenever we are uncomfortable, need a diaper changed, are hungry, thirsty, hot, cold, scared, or lonely. Yet relatively quickly we develop more sophisticated strategies and tactics for getting what we want. We learn from experience what works, and what doesn't. We mirror the behavior of our parents. We observe techniques from siblings, school friends, books, television, movies, and the internet. Bit by bit the various inputs and experiences form our opinions, beliefs, and motivations. We may believe that by the time we reach adulthood these beliefs, opinions, and behaviors are rational, sensible, and mature approaches to life. And on the surface, they may be, but it is worth remembering that we designed these strategies and tactics as children, from the age of about two. There are, therefore, some flaws in the foundations of our psyches.

If we were made to feel safe and secure as a baby, the chances are that we end up trusting the world, see it primarily as a friendly place, and have a healthy appetite for exploration, discovery, and risk based on our sense that everything is ultimately okay. If we were ignored as babies, we tend to feel insecure, and our foundational approach to the world is one of caution, distrust, and an aversion to exploration or risk because at the end of the day things are not okay. These are only a couple of the ways in which our deep-seated approaches toward life get skewed by the interpretation of an infant. Most of these profound building blocks of our personalities are so instinctive that we are not even aware of them as options; it is just 'who we are.'

I could have approached my dinner with Sally by reminding myself that the purpose was not to create a perfect meal but to have an enjoyable evening with my girlfriend. I could have recognized that the stress I felt about my life was self-generated and that there is no committee of people disapproving of me, except in my mind. I could have realized that my sense of the appropriate time to eat was completely fictional, based again on a projection of what 'other people would think,' rather than on what was okay for us. I'm a reasonably rational and self-aware person who has the ability to see all of those things, yet I still blew it. The problem is that the base operating system on top of which all that rationality sits is faulty. I can operate well enough in the world to have a career, a house, friends, and some money in the bank, but every so often it reveals its shortcomings. Stress brings the flaws to light.

My father is an amazing parent for whom I am incredibly grateful. He provided security for my family, he was a stabilizing force in an otherwise chaotic home, and he is generous, caring and loving. Yet, not surprisingly, he did not completely pull off the impossible – namely raising kids without hang-ups. Part of his parenting style (or to be fair to him, my sense of his parenting style) was to protect me from making mistakes. There wasn't a great deal of praise for everyday achievements, only corrections when I screwed up. I realize this is great parenting compared to what many people get, but it resulted in a flaw in my operating system.

As a child, I was trying to make sense of the world. I was building a psychological map for who I was, how to survive, and how to get love. Each interaction serves as a disproportionately large input into how that map gets built. I had no way of seeing a bigger picture or rationalizing that his criticisms were his demonstrations of love; that he was protecting me, and I misinterpreted what was going on. Thanks to a bunch of therapy I eventually came to see how I had ended up terrified of making mistakes and how I equated criticism with being unworthy of love. As a young child, I made the error of believing that I had to be perfect, I had to avoid mistakes in order to avoid criticism, in order to be valued and loved. This is how the child interpreted the input.

Even with therapy, it is still how my operating system works today. At my core, deep down, I remain terrified of criticism. I find it incredibly hard to do things that might go wrong because the underlying operating system believes I will get criticized and then be unworthy of love. I know it is very rare for anyone to like criticism, but for some of us, it is more like a paralyzing phobia than something unpleasant. Being aware that this is how my deep down self views the world has helped me see and understand the behavior, but awareness of it has not fixed the programming. Arguing with myself that I'm behaving irrationally is almost literally like arguing with a two year old. My rational self may be right, but the two year old doesn't care.

So, on this Saturday as I was feeling particularly aware of how imperfect my life was, and that things were not working out as I'd hoped, my inner child started getting scared. Even though the purpose of dinner was to enjoy the evening with Sally, I started to get terrified that she was going to disapprove of the food, of the meal for being so late, of me for being so disorganized, of me in general. If my rational self were in control, I would have been able to have perspective, to see the priority and adjust. However, the rational self often loses control when under stress. Under stress, the two year old's operating system took over. I was running scared and behaving like a kid trying to avoid being told off.

Our psyches have flawed foundations, which makes it challenging to manage our minds and our behavior. In addition to that, even our rational mind is often conflicted. We want a sense of safety, security, and certainty, of knowing what's what and having some control over our destiny. Yet at the same time, we want diversity, variety, excitement, and the unexpected. We want to be recognized as individuals, to be different, to be special, unique, and yet we want to belong, to be normal, to fit in, to be part of something bigger than ourselves. Many of our wants and needs are contradictory, and we are constantly trying to find the right balance for ourselves. When a friend tells me a story that he wants me to keep secret, I want to respect that trust and be a loyal friend. But when I am at a dinner party, and I think the story would make everyone laugh, I want to tell it. Whether I do or not, depends on which desire wins out, my desire to be trustworthy, or my desire to be popular and liked in the short term. Which one wins, in turn, depends on how much I need my ego stroked in that moment, how I feel about my friend, what was drilled into me as a child about keeping secrets, and how committed I am to the idea of hard principles (never tell), rather than a situational weighing of outcomes (maybe it's okay this time).

Philosophers, psychologists, sociologists, anthropologists, and other social scientists have tried to model the conflicting aspects of human behavior by reducing it down to a few organizing principles that make sense of why we behave the way we do. An early proposal suggested we were made up of four elements: fire, earth, wind, and water. Our needs, wants, motivations, and behaviors could be understood by the balance of these. Modern models might include Abraham Maslow's Hierarchy of Needs, Freud's model of our psyche as being an ego, id, and superego, or Carl Jung's hypothesis regarding the four ways in which humans view the world from which the Myers-Briggs model was derived. Many of these models are useful. Yet the plethora and ever increasing number of them is a good indicator that none serves as a complete explanation.

Humans are complex creatures. Literature and art are filled with explorations of the infinite numbers of ways in which our lives can manifest. Good art speaks to us because even though we are all unique packages of needs, wants, motivations, and behaviors we can still relate to each other's unique packages.

In a relationship, you are trying to put together two complex packages of needs, wants, motivations, and behaviors. It should not be surprising that sometimes it doesn't work. It is more surprising that it ever works. Between you, you have two maps of the world whose foundations were built by infants based on a few experiences and no perspective. We are internally conflicted individuals who aren't particularly great at working out what makes us happy, let alone trying to work out how to keep two people happy at the same time. It is easy to see why small things, like how fast the other person is driving, can cause tension long before you get to more significant challenges.

Meditation and Conflict

As I unfortunately demonstrated at the beginning of this chapter, meditation is not going to turn you into a saint who never loses it or behaves badly. What it can do is help you behave badly less often, and when you do lose it, you can get it back far more quickly and limit the damage of your bad behavior.

In awareness meditation, you sit and focus, very commonly on your breathing. You become aware of your thoughts as the mind wanders, you develop awareness of the sensations in your body, you notice how you feel emotionally, and eventually become sensitive to changes as they are occurring in your body. On one hand, this is a training in bringing your awareness into the present moment rather than flitting around in the past or future inside your head. On the other hand, this is an incredibly useful training in starting to become far more sensitive to what is going on from moment to moment, not only in meditation, but throughout your day.

I recently attended a charity works project where a number of people got together to paint a children's day care center. I showed up willing to help out in any way I could. I was paired up with someone I didn't know and sent to prepare the bathrooms. We were asked to put up plastic sheeting so that when people came in to clean their brushes and rollers, they wouldn't splatter the bathroom with paint. I've done enough painting in my own house to know there is a trick to getting the plastic to sit flat and for it not to tear off the walls as soon as someone treads on it. The guy I was working with did not know this and started doing it exactly the wrong way. Almost immediately my childhood programming kicked in, and I could feel myself getting upset about the fact that we were doing it all wrong. My instinct was to get him out of the way, to take control, and get it done properly. This time though, I noticed the feelings as they arose. I could feel the anxiety, frustration, and fear as they poured through me. This time I saw them for what they were. I was able to pause and assess whether my programming was helpful at that moment. It wasn't. The bigger picture was that we were there to work collaboratively on this project. It didn't need to be done quickly or correctly the first time. I took a breath and smiled to myself about my unhelpful instincts. I let my colleague have a go, let him get it wrong, and then gently suggested a different way we might go about it. The whole exercise took us maybe ten minutes longer than if I had jumped in and taken control, but the result was better. We bonded, had a nice moment together doing the work, and I felt better about not allowing myself to be the jerk I can be.

If you are human, you are going to experience frustration, anger, nervousness, jealousy, and sadness from time to time. It is also part of the human dilemma that you are most likely to experience these when you are around your significant other, or with your immediate family. Meditation isn't going to make you immune from feeling the full range of emotions. What it can do is help you see these powerful forces as they arise. That gives you the ability in that moment to investigate what is going on within you and to then decide what you want to do about it.

Managing Conflict When You're in It

It's great to have a plan to help avoid conflict, but sometimes that plan fails, and you find yourself in the middle of it. They've said something, you've said something, someone's got hurt, tensions have risen. The meditation practice to this point has failed to prevent a fight. It can still help.

Awareness meditation starts by focusing on the breath, and then your mind wanders. The instruction is always the same – when you notice your mind has wandered, gently bring it back to the breath. This can sometimes seem boring, repetitive, and pointless. When you are in the middle of a fight is when it pays dividends to have stuck with it.

When passions are swirling, it is hard to pause, to notice where your mind is racing, and to become aware of your powerful feelings. It is not easy, but with training it is possible. If you have repeatedly trained yourself to notice where your mind is, from moment to moment in meditation, you have a chance in the middle of the fight to notice what's going on. This moment of awareness can give you the opportunity to pause, recognizing that no matter how strong your emotions are right now, there is a chance, a tiny chance perhaps, but a chance nevertheless, that the course of action you are determined to take, or the thing you are determined to say, may, possibly, not be the best thing in the long run. Limiting the damage here can make a big difference to the next few hours, days, or even to the long-term trajectory of your relationship. It isn't easy, but regular meditation practice does give you the possibility of pausing in the middle of it all and seeing what is going on. If that happens, then try to ask yourself a few questions.

"What are you feeling right now?" To which the answer might be,

"Angry. Frustrated. Hurt. Disappointed." Then,

"Why are you angry, frustrated, nervous, or whatever?"

"Because they're wrong," or "They're being stupid," or "They are so thoughtless," or "This is bad."

These are possibilities of course, but these are not always relevant or helpful explanations. Even if the person you are dealing with is wrong, why is that making you upset? What is at stake for you? Why does it matter? If you can see yourself getting upset, you can investigate and get to the bottom of it. You may be perfectly justified in your anger, jealousy, sadness, or whatever, but you may not be. If you are, then the question is how can you now act most sensibly or constructively. Perhaps your partner did something or said something very hurtful. You can, of course, retaliate in kind and hurt them back. Or you can see that you are hurt, and you can choose not to retaliate. You can ask yourself whether they really meant to hurt you. If they did ... that's a bigger issue and probably needs some work to find out what that's about and what you want to do. Alternatively, they may merely be being stupid, which many of us are from time to time. If you retaliate, you are going to keep the battle going and are likely to cause more damage instead of holding fire. You can pause. Perhaps take a breath and allow your emotions to settle slightly. Then you gauge where the other person is mentally and emotionally, and try to think about where you want the conflict to go.

In another situation where we notice ourselves animated with powerful emotions, we can pause and ask whether this is really about what's going on in front of us, or if this is part of your childhood programming of defensiveness, self-esteem issues, or whatever. Is it part of theirs? In my case, during the dinner, I missed this, but could have seen that my anxiety was really about my deep-seated but unhelpful and erroneous belief that I have to be perfect. It had no basis in what was going on in front of me. I was also carrying my stress about what had happened earlier in my day into the dinner, and I was acting out over that rather than the fact that the parsnips were going to be done too quickly. Often if we can catch ourselves we can see that our emotions may not have anything to do with what's going on in front of us; they're reacting to a different situation altogether.

Another helpful question you can ask is how much you are trying to be right. If you ask people what is their objective in a heated discussion, they may say they are trying to explain their point of view, and perhaps that they are also trying to understand the other person's point of view. However, one of the strongest psychological forces within humans is simply the desire to be right. Once the fight starts, the point of the fight can get lost very quickly, and it becomes only about winning.

One of the only things stronger than wanting to be right is the sibling to this desire, the fear of being wrong. People will defend their position almost to the death rather than be wrong. Even if they know they are wrong, it feels better to continue to defend the indefensible rather than capitulate. When people say that they have no problem admitting when they are wrong, it is only true when they don't care about the subject. Give them something they hold to be true, whether it is about religion, politics, ethics, morality, or whether their child is a good person, and they will not back down without a fight, even when the evidence is blatant that they're wrong.

The desire to be right and fear of being wrong are very, very powerful. They cause families to stop talking to each other, spouses to break up, and can turn friends into enemies. In the moment when you become aware of heightened emotions one of the most useful questions you can ask is whether this is motivating your position right now. Are you trying to be right? Are you trying to avoid being wrong? Are you trying to get them to admit they're wrong? (By the way – don't do this, it is futile: they'd probably rather die than do this.) You can also try to remember the bigger picture, and try to see the other person's point of view. Perhaps ask yourself what is available if you let go of your position. What do you really want to get out of this interaction? Is being right more important to you than your relationship? In the heat of the moment, it is incredible how often the immediate answer to this is 'Yes.' But take a breath. Pause. Maybe then ask if there is a compromise that could save everything. Sometimes there is.

HALT

HALT is an acronym talked about in addiction programs to help people become aware of when they are liable to make bad decisions or act in destructive ways. It stands for Hungry, Angry, Lonely, or Tired. In a conflict situation, it is worth bearing in mind your state of being, and the state of being of the person you're fighting with. Are you hungry? You are probably angry or at least moving in that direction which is why you're asking this question, but what else is going on? Are you, or are they feeling isolated, unsupported, ignored, not listened to, or lonely? Are you, or are they tired? Most of us are not at our best when tired. If you are aware enough to notice your emotions, ask whether this is about your state of mind. If any of these are true, it is likely that this is causing the fight, rather than whatever it is you're ostensibly fighting about.

Tactics Are Useless Without Awareness

These tactics are available in books or seminars on conflict handling. The knowledge seems helpful for those who haven't previously heard it. But the advice assumes that people are able to be aware of what is going on in the moment. Without that awareness, the knowledge is useless. I have seen advice explaining to people that they need to be more aware of what they are feeling as they are feeling it. This advice is also completely useless. Either you are aware, or you're not in any given moment, and if you're not aware then you're certainly not going to be able to suddenly say, "Oh, I should try being aware in this moment." Awareness is not something you can turn on when you want. It needs training. This is one of the reasons people like meditation. If you meditate, your awareness gets developed. You notice more. Not everything, and not every time, but a lot more often. Once you develop awareness, then you have the power to use these and other techniques for preventing conflict, or for handling it more skillfully as it occurs.

This Is Great, but This Is Work

The violinist Jascha Heifetz was once asked whether he practiced every day. It seemed he was so skillful that perhaps he no longer needed to. His response was that he did.

"If I don't practice one day, I know it; two days, the critics know it; three days, the public knows it."

Meditation training is like this. If you go to a class once, it will probably make you feel better, but it is like going to the gym once. It is better than not going but won't do you much good in the long term. If you go occasionally, it is again, better than not going at all. But if you go every day you start to develop real strength, fitness, and flexibility. I maintain that meditation is a remarkable practice with incredible benefits. But, I regret to admit, it does take work, diligence, and persistence to see some of those benefits. In my meditation practice, when I am practicing regularly, most things tend to go well. But if I drop it, or cut my meditations short there is a difference. Like Heifetz, if I miss a day, I notice. If I miss two days, Sally notices (and not so subtly asks whether I got my meditation in recently). If I miss three days, everyone notices.

CHAPTER FOUR

The Pursuit of Happiness

I am a bit of a curmudgeon. I'm about to tell you about happiness, and I'm going to suggest that meditation is helpful, but I have to start by admitting I'm a pretty grumpy guy. I wish I were a glass is half full kind of person, but I'm not, and I'm also grumpy about the fact that I'm not. I regularly see what's wrong with things instead of what's right. Meditation has helped me be less grumpy, but it hasn't fixed me.

One of the things that I get grumpy about is our education system. When I was in school, I was taught a bunch of completely useless things. I felt like I didn't study anything truly important. I learned formulas for how gas expands and contracts with temperature and pressure (Boyle's Law), and can remember the name of a chemical that absorbs oxygen (pyrogallic acid), and I learned a bunch of calculus. "Tempus erat quo prima quies mortalibus aegris" is etched into my memory as line 268 of Virgil's *Aeneid Book II* because the only way I was ever going to pass Latin was to memorize the text and its translation. I have never had any use for any of those things in my life other than passing exams and getting me into university.

On the other hand, none of the most important aspects of life such as relationships, finances, careers, love, sex, managing emotions, or parenting were covered. Not a single class. Go figure. Surely happiness, the most fundamental of human pursuits would have been covered, but no, it was not. In fact, much of my school experience was, instead, an education in unhappiness. But thank goodness I can also remember the next line from Virgil's *Aeneid* – "incipit et dono divum gratissima serpit." See, I told you I was a curmudgeon.

How would I have taught happiness? We could have started with the early philosophers and looked at their different theories. Perhaps we would then have looked at the guidance of different religious traditions and their proposals on how to live a life. We could have explored the pros and cons of the popular ways in which people pursue happiness in the modern world such as money, sex, power, love, or fame. Perhaps there would have been no final answers as to what makes someone happy, but at least we could have looked at theories and options, thought about it, discussed it, and argued different points of view.

Today, thanks to a psychologist named Marty Seligman, you would have a big advantage in setting a curriculum over when I was in school. He tells a story about how he was, like me, a pretty grumpy guy. One day he was gardening, and his young daughter was annoying him by playing with the weeds he'd pulled out. At some point, he snapped at her, and she ran off in tears. The story goes that after a while she came back out to talk to him. She suggested that she had whined a great deal until her fifth birthday but that she decided on that day she would stop whining, and that she hadn't done so since. She said it was the hardest thing she'd ever done, but if she could stop whining, then he could stop being such a grump. Her statement struck him. He thought about it and wondered if that was true. Could he stop being such a grump, or was his general level of happiness, or grumpiness fixed?

That moment in Seligman's garden was the spark that kindled what is now known as Positive Psychology. He decided to start to research happiness. He pitched his ideas to the American Psychological Association and was elected President in 1998 with the platform to start to dedicate more time and research for looking at human well-being rather than just mental pathologies.

There have been many findings since then about what contributes to human happiness. One piece of research was a Harvard study by Matt Killingsworth and Dan Gilbert. The results were published in November 2010 under the title "A Wandering Mind is an Unhappy Mind."

Killingsworth and Gilbert built an app for people's smartphones, and thousands of people downloaded it. The app would query people at random points of the day and ask them three questions: how happy they were, what they were doing, and whether they were thinking about their current activity or about something else that was pleasant, neutral, or unpleasant. What they discovered was that people were distracted and not focused on what they were doing about 47% of the time. In fact, the only activity where people were focused more than 70% of the time was sex. What they also discovered was that the correlation of happiness was not the activity itself, but merely whether the subject was focused on the activity at hand or not. One of the aspects of human minds is that they wander, but the wandering mind is not a happy one.

Think about it for a second. What are the things that you are happiest doing? It might be meeting friends, going to the movies, reading a book, doing the crossword, hiking, working out, going to a sporting event, listening to music, watching TV, or having sex. All of the things you enjoy doing the most are things that by their very nature hold your attention strongly. We may think we are fully focused because we are enjoying them. Or, is it, as the research suggests, that we enjoy them *because* they hold our attention?

When I am feeling sorry for myself or otherwise miserable, my default behavior is to put on a movie or binge watch a TV show. It works. At least in the short term I don't feel the anxiety, sadness, anger, depression, jealousy, or frustration that I might have been feeling beforehand. I am distracted from my own mind by virtue of having it pulled into the storyline of what's in front of me. The more thrilling or compelling the story, the better I am distracted from my own life.

The Mind Can Be Our Best Friend, or Our Worst Enemy

As a friend, our mind is who we think we are. It is our personality, our thoughts, our beliefs, our opinions. It helps us navigate the world, allows us to interact with our friends, family, and loved ones, as well as helps us deal with work colleagues and neighbors. It reminds us to take out the trash, to get our taxes done, to wake up at certain times, to try to eat healthily, and to remember to call our mothers.

As an enemy, our mind is constantly reminding us we are not good enough. It compares us to other people who are 'better' than we are. It looks at what's wrong with our lives. It creates catastrophic fantasies about the impending crash of our plane, about the deaths of people closest to us, of terrorism, or home invasion. Less catastrophic but also unhelpful concerns include worrying what everyone will think about us, about our lover leaving us, or about how every headache, lump, or cold probably means we have cancer.

The wandering mind is an unhappy mind. The research from Killingsworth and Gilbert has been reinforced by looking at brain activity with EEGs and fMRIs that suggest that when we are wandering around in our mind, thinking about ourselves and our lives, what the scientists refer to as ruminating, it takes place in the part of the brain associated with sadder and more depressive states of mind. When we are completely focused on something, the activity takes place in the part of the brain associated with happiness, joy, and well-being. There is more research to be done, but we know a great deal more about happiness now than we have ever known. What does this knowledge tell us?

Happiness can be a choice. We have options. We can keep ourselves busy and focused. If we are so busy that we don't give our minds a chance to wander we are not unhappy. This doesn't completely work of course because it is hard to be fully focused all the time, but nevertheless, it appears to support the theory that busy people literally don't have time to be unhappy. There is an argument that some daydreaming allows for creativity and inspiration, so if you are fully focused all the time, how do you get new ideas?

Here is where I make the pitch for meditation. The practice of meditation, particularly that of awareness meditation is a training in focus. It is also a training in noticing when you are not focused. I feel as though when people read the findings of Killingsworth and Gilbert that they say, "Ah, interesting, I should be more focused on what I'm doing. Okay, I'll do that." But it isn't that easy. If you could do that, meditation would be easy. You would sit down and say, "I'm going to focus on my breath." You would sit and be focused on the breath. When we sit down, that's not what happens. You can have all the determination you want, but it won't work. Your mind wanders. That's what it does. Meditation develops the ability to see where your mind is at any given moment, and then the ability to be focused, or not, whenever you want. If you want to daydream, ponder your life, or to try to solve problems – you can. If you want to be focused, you can. Meditation is the training to help you to choose what to do with your mind.

Focus Is Good, Where You Are Focused Is Better

So, I'm a curmudgeon and generally grumpy, but thanks to meditation I can choose to be focused, and while I'm focused I'm not unhappy. It's a good start, but starting to notice where you are focused is even more helpful in determining your happiness.

Some of the most inspiring people giving TED talks are those people who have every right to be miserable but are not. These are people who have been dealt a rough hand of cards by life. What is inspiring to us is that they have every justification for feeling sorry for themselves or for being miserable, but they are not. They have somehow managed to find joy in spite of everything. The opposite of these people are those who seem to have everything and yet remain angry, frustrated and sad. The single simplest difference between the two groups of people is the way they look at the world.

If you ask the question what is wrong with your life, you will always have lots of answers, no matter how rich, healthy, or lucky you are. I remember years ago being in San Francisco and hearing someone complaining about how they had just got their BMW washed, and then it rained – "Can you believe that!"

Alternatively, if you ask the question – what is right with your life, and you try a little bit, you can also have lots of answers. Which question are you asking? Where is your focus? Of course, it makes sense to be aware of what you can do to improve your situation, but when you are perpetually focused on what is wrong, you will be miserable. If you are generally focused on what is right, gratitude arises, and you will be happy.

Where you put your focus is the difference between being happy and being miserable. Which is perhaps interesting knowledge, but is useless unless you can develop the awareness of where your focus is in the first place, and then have the ability to change your focus when it isn't somewhere that helps. Meditation helps you become aware of what's going on in your mind, where you are focused and gives you the ability to see if that's where you want to be focused. It trains you in moving your focus back to where you want it to be.

In breath meditation, you are continually refocusing on the breath from wherever you went in your distractions. In your life, you can notice you have started to focus on things that are unhelpful, and you can then choose to change that focus to something more helpful. It doesn't change the circumstances of your life, but inspirational individuals in terrible situations show that your happiness is not dictated by your circumstances, it is in how you choose to look at them. Meditation is the training that allows you to change your focus.

Compassion Training

Breath meditation is useful in developing our awareness of where our mind has gone and training us in the skill to move it wherever we want, but there is another type of meditation that is perhaps even more useful. Compassion meditation is a training that can change where our mind goes in the first place because it changes us at our core. I'll go into more detail later about how to do it, but whereas awareness meditation helps your mind, compassion meditation helps your heart. As great as your mind is, your heart is more powerful. Everything changes when you start to exercise your love, generosity, and compassion.

In the situation where a driver does something selfish or dangerous in front of you, you might get annoyed or even angry. You might explode in your mind that they're an idiot, or that their behavior is exactly what is wrong with society today. Thanks to awareness meditation you might become aware of your thoughts, your anger, your adrenaline and see it for what it is. You can then decide what you want to do, whether you want to continue down that road of being upset, or choose to put your mind somewhere else, recognizing that getting upset is only affecting you. With compassion meditation training, your mind can start to go in a different direction. You're not going to stop caring about what's wrong in the world, but your default reactions are going to change. You might still get a stab of frustration that someone drove dangerously, but the default reaction can change because you recognize that they are human, fallible, and yes, maybe selfish - as you are sometimes. Your default reaction can change to consider that maybe they are in a legitimate hurry, perhaps they are racing to the hospital to visit someone, perhaps they are late for an important meeting. It might not be true, but the immediate reaction changes, and then you still get to decide what you want to do about it.

An argument against this approach is that maybe the bad driver is being stupid, or reckless. Perhaps they are, but you don't have control over that. You only have a choice of how you are going to react to the world. One habitual reaction is going to make you upset and angry. Or the other habitual reaction causes barely a blip on your well-being. However, it isn't a choice in the moment. The choice happens beforehand. You choose every day whether to work on how you are going to see the world, or not.

Do you want to be subject to anger, frustration, and disappointment every time something happens that you don't like? Or would you like to try to develop that side of you that is more like a Martin Luther King, Gandhi, Nelson Mandela, or the Dalai Lama? These people were not pushovers that didn't try to change what was wrong in the world. But they nevertheless approached the world from a place of generosity, compassion, and love. Some people will argue they were as effective as they were *because* they approached the world from compassion, and not from anger. You and I may never be as good at it as they were, but we can get better, and closer to their examples. It takes work. Compassion meditation is that work.

Easing Suffering

In 1997 my meditation teacher encouraged students with an interest to start teaching. Teaching is a great way to improve your own practice. Teaching is also rewarding in its own right, and teaching meditation is particularly so because people love it and are always very grateful for the classes. But teaching can also be intimidating and I procrastinated for a couple of years before starting.

I hadn't read every book I could on the subject, and I was sure I didn't know enough. I was nervous that no one would show up and I was also nervous that too many people would show up. I lacked confidence in my ability to communicate the techniques or to inspire people to try it. My inability to see these fears for what they were was not very impressive for someone who was meditating, let alone someone who was supposed to be teaching meditation. It was only at the urging of a friend that I started. He was running an acting studio and felt it might be valuable for his students to help them become more present, and less in their heads. I rented a space and put up some posters to advertise. To my relief and horror, some people showed up.

After a few classes, I was still very unsure as to whether I was offering anything of value. Then something happened that helped me realize my class didn't have to be brilliant to be worthwhile. I had just started my fourth or fifth class when a dirty and very bedraggled, possibly homeless guy came in. He sat at the back and never seemed to fully engage with the session. He couldn't sit still and made a lot of noise whenever he changed his position. He would also make a lot of exasperated noises while I was talking, and even during the meditations themselves. At the end of the class, I was unsure what he was going to say as he approached me. His eyes were darting left and right, and he looked very uncomfortable. I was about to apologize and offer him his money back when he said, "Thanks for that class Justyn. I don't think I'm going to have to kill myself now."

I was thrown and didn't really know what to say. I asked him to explain, and he let me know that he'd been an addict of alcohol and drugs for many years but had recently given it up. He'd taken to alcohol and drugs as a way of silencing the voice in his head. It wasn't so much that he was schizophrenic, rather that his own inner critic was very loud and relentlessly putting him down. He'd self-medicated for years, but that was killing him, so he'd given it up. However, without the drugs and alcohol the voice in his head was so strong, and making him so miserable he didn't know what to do. He said he'd more or less resigned himself to suicide as his only option. At an AA meeting, someone had talked about meditation and with nothing to lose he decided to check out my class. Despite his fidgeting, he said he'd managed to get a little bit of peace from his own mind during the meditations, and he thought maybe he wasn't going to have to kill himself after all. He had hope that maybe if he could learn this meditation thing, he would be able to keep going. I never saw him again, and I don't know what happened. I hope he found some peace.

This chapter is about happiness and meditation. Meditation makes you happier. But I don't think meditation even has to make you happier to be worthwhile. The level of unhappiness in our society today is chronic. A Medco report in 2011 suggested that more than one in five women in the U.S. over the age of twenty use anti-depressants. We lose more people to drug overdose than car crashes or gun deaths. The political climate around the world is one of anger and frustration. In the United States, we are richer than any society in history, and yet we are miserable. Meditation may be able to make you happier, but happiness is not even the bar meditation would need to cross to be worthwhile. If it can help people be less miserable, that would be enough.

We may not be driven to the extreme of the man in my class, yet most of us also wrestle with that critic in our heads. We tend to believe it is useful. It is driving us to be better. It says 'helpful' things like "You don't know enough, you're not clever enough, you're not pretty enough, not thin enough." "You don't work hard enough, you're not funny enough, not creative enough, not good enough." And we listen. We see our faults, and we believe that we need to keep beating ourselves up. Some of us turn to therapy, to prescription medications, or to other forms of medication. I encourage anyone to try therapy, and I am absolutely in favor of people using psychiatry with all its pharmaceutical interventions when necessary. However, I also believe and am backed up by scientific research, that meditation also helps. It helps those that aren't in therapy or on medication and helps many in conjunction with therapy, or medication. It helps us take a break from ourselves, without necessarily having to reach for a pill, the bottle, or something stronger.

A Work in Progress

I am still a grouch sometimes. I still indulge in self-pity. I still get miserable. I compare myself to others and feel like a failure. I still beat myself up about my lack of discipline, my lack of success, about my weight, about my hair having fallen out, about my selfishness, and lack of talent. But I do it a great deal less than I used to.

I am happier most of the day, most days, but still have a tendency to see the emptiness of the glass rather than its fullness. Despite feeling much better than I used to, I want perfection, and I see the empty part of the glass as the fact that meditation has not delivered perfection. I can see that my glass is probably three quarters full now, yet I still get frustrated that it's a quarter empty. But I don't do that as much as I used to.

I haven't 'fixed' myself, but I am more accepting of good rather than perfect. I wish I could tell you meditation will work completely, that you'll be happy all the time, but I can't. I can only tell you it can make you happier than you are, and suggest that if you want perfection, perhaps you can try this to get you closer than you are today. It might also help you let go of perfection. I'm still holding out for the extra quarter of the glass, but I suspect that the last quarter probably fills up when you stop trying to fill it up.

Meditation, like any other practice in well-being (exercise, health, etc.), is not a one-and-done solution, but something that you have to engage in regularly to reap its full benefits. I wish that meditation was something you could occasionally do and get all the benefits. It isn't. When I'm not meditating regularly, I revert to being more of a grump. When I meditate regularly, I am happier.

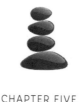

CHAPTER FIVE

Health

Change Your Relationship with Your Body

It is a Wednesday night at a church in New Jersey. Around fifty people are sitting upright with their eyes closed. I am guiding them through a "body scan" awareness meditation. I invite them to notice and become aware of the different parts of their body. We start by getting a sense of the whole body, and then move the attention to specific parts. The big toe of the left foot. The second toe on the left foot. It goes on. I ask people to notice where they can sense pressure on their foot from the floor, or from their shoe. We do the whole of the left leg and then switch to the right. We notice knees, hips, and then move to the torso, and eventually get to the arms, the neck, the head. As we move our attention around the body, I ask people to notice what is going on, to notice the sensations without judging or starting a conversation in their heads about the sensations. If there are aches and pains, notice them and perhaps look closely to see what shape and texture the aches and pains take, but try to avoid talking to yourself about the pain being wrong. For this exercise, we are simply developing our awareness of what is present in our bodies, without commentary. It takes about twenty minutes, and then I ask everyone to take a deep breath, relax, and open their eyes. After a minute or so I ask them how they found the exercise.

The feedback for this exercise is fairly consistent. Some find it to be very relaxing. They say it gets them to slow down, to get out of their thinking mind, and to pay attention to the body. Some people comment on how surprised they are at the quantity of information being communicated by their bodies that they are usually not aware of, or are ignoring. Many people, however, don't like the exercise.

The reason many people don't like the exercise is because they don't like getting in touch with their bodies. Their bodies hurt. For some people, their bodies hurt all the time and getting them to pay attention is only making them more aware of their hurt. Or their bodies don't work as well as they wished they did. Digestive problems, breathing problems, allergies, sensitivities, anxieties, and addictions are held in the body causing frustration. For some, it is that their body reminds them they are getting older in a way that our mind never does. In our minds, we are still 25, or 16, or 7, but our bodies know how old we are and putting our attention there reminds us. Many feel as though their body has let them down. It has gained more weight than they wanted, it doesn't work as well as it used to, or it doesn't look the way they want it to look.

I don't particularly enjoy teaching this class because I know how difficult people's relationships with their body can be. Yet I know the value of this exercise and what can lie on the other side.

The first thing about meditating on the body and the physical sensations is that it gets us out of our heads. If our attention is focused on the feelings in the body, we are not thinking about tomorrow, yesterday, or worrying about some issue in our lives. The information the body is sending is always in real-time, so it is a powerful tool for helping people get into the present and to start to understand what that means.

The second thing is to help people become aware of this relationship they have with their body. It is often a dysfunctional one.

Imagine an unhappily married couple that has been together for decades. They aren't going to leave each other at this point, but they clearly don't like each other anymore. Every interaction is a battle. There is relentless sniping and complaining. They resent each other, and they resent the circumstances that have led them to this situation. You might think that they should leave each other but for whatever reasons, leaving would be even worse than the prospect of staying together. Neither is going to change, yet they keep trying to convince the other to do so and keep resenting them for not doing it. That is more or less the relationship many of us have with our body. Many of us see it as a disappointment at best, and at worst as an enemy that we are stuck with.

Imagine for a second that your body was someone you knew, a person you were in a relationship with, and put yourself in their shoes. What would it be like to be living under that level of disappointment and resentment? What would happen if you became aware of your attitude towards them and changed it? What would happen if you changed your focus from what is wrong with them, to what is right with them? What would happen if you loved them exactly as they are – what would that do for you, what would that do for them, and what might change as a result?

This is easy to say. It is surprisingly difficult to do. We have deep-seated resentments that our bodies are imperfect, defective, ugly, or fat. In order to change your attitude, you have to be aware of your attitude in the first place. Most people aren't until it gets pointed out. How do you feel about your body? There are hopefully many things you like about it, but what are your complaints, and how do you feel about those complaints?

The ability to notice where you are focused, and then to change that focus, is such an important aspect of meditation. In respect to our bodies, are we focused on what is wrong with our body, or on what is right with our body? When we are focused on what is wrong, the answers may be correct, but they are unhelpful if they make us unhappy with ourselves and resentful. If we focus on what is right, those answers are no more or less correct than those we have for what is wrong, but focusing on those answers can generate feelings of gratitude and even awe.

Your body is an extraordinary instrument, literally millions of years in the making. In any given moment it is performing thousands of complex tasks. It is absorbing oxygen and getting rid of carbon dioxide. It is making new blood, pumping it around your body, and getting rid of old toxins. It is digesting, breaking down food into constituent parts and distributing them so that you can use them when you need them. It is performing hundreds of chemical balancing acts to keep you alive with exactly the right pH levels and the right concentrations of hundreds of other hormones and minerals. It is absorbing an extraordinary amount of information and filtering that information automatically so that you are aware of only what you need to be aware of. It is highly coordinated, even those of us who aren't as highly coordinated as others. We can still walk, run, drive cars, cook, watch movies, listen to music, throw things in roughly the right direction, and catch other things – at least some of the time. We can meet new people and process vast quantities of subliminal information to decide if we like them, if we trust them, if we are attracted to them, or if we don't like them. We can also pick up if they like us, if they trust us, if they are attracted to us.

Take vision as one example. Light waves are hitting the back of our retina – a curved, but essentially two-dimensional surface. Our optic nerve is taking information about those light waves back to our brain which then creates a picture in our brain based on the light that hit the back of the eye. Those pictures, what we 'see,' have been converted from light hitting the two dimensional surface at the back of our eye and now appear as three dimensional objects in our mind with texture, color, movement, weight, and speed. All this happens in real time. Our bodies may not be perfect, but they are miraculous.

It's not that you shouldn't critique what's wrong, but how would you criticize the imperfections if you were talking to a best friend? Would you get angry with them for not being perfect? Or would you ask questions and work out together what you might do to improve a situation? If you see them for what they are rather than for what they are not, perhaps you might even give them a break for their imperfections. You would at least be a lot happier even if they didn't change, recognizing them as a friend, as someone who is doing extraordinary things for you, even if they aren't doing everything you want.

Awareness meditation training, like watching the breath, or doing a body scan can help us see our approach and our focus, and can train us in being able to move our focus and hence our attitude and approach towards our body to something else if we want.

If we apply compassion meditation toward our body, we can see even more dramatic shifts in our attitude towards our bodies. The training helps open our heart, our generosity, and our love. We tend to believe we are loving people, but how much do we practice that? Do we practice our capacity for love more than we practice our capacity for cynicism, judgment, and resentment? Compassion training gives us a chance to change that balance. It enables us to love ourselves and others more easily, even things we don't 'like' much, such as our bodies.

If you start to love your body, or at the very least start to like your body, it may, or may not change. But you will change how you treat it. If you see the cheeseburger on the menu, and you really want the cheeseburger, but you know that your body doesn't want the cheeseburger, do you still order it? Maybe you still do, but maybe not as often. Maybe you start to try to treat yourself better. Maybe you remember to give it some water, sleep, gentle exercise, or fruit. Again, this is easier said than done. I'm sure many of you 'know' you're supposed to treat your body better, but it's not a priority. The healthy choices can always start tomorrow. Like being nicer to your spouse can always start when they start being nicer to you. Meditation, both awareness and compassion training, can make the difference so that you start being nicer to yourself today. You'll be happier, you'll treat your body better, and it might react to that kindness by becoming healthier, fitter, or in less pain.

Stress

A major motivation for writing this book was in reaction to the widely-held belief that meditation is for stress relief. Meditation is about so much more than stress relief. Stress relief is just a nice, ancillary benefit of meditation but it is certainly not its main purpose. Nevertheless, I recognize that stress reduction is a major reason people come to meditation. Many people are over-stressed, and chronic stress is exceptionally bad for you. Meditation works in alleviating stress and helping us manage stressful situations better. So let's look at stress in more detail and see what's going on when you meditate.

Stress is a complex topic. Scientists don't tend to use the word stress because it doesn't mean to them what it means to us. What we think of as stress, they see as merely one end of a continuum of physiological arousal. At one end of the scale, scientists see complete relaxation, with a slower pulse rate, calmer brain activity, and a negligible presence of adrenaline or related hormones. Then there is some 'arousal,' which could appear as anticipation, energy, or excitement. Try to remember that feeling you got as a kid before your birthday. There were elevated levels of hope and expectation. Not what we'd think of as stress, but from a scientist's point of view this is part of the continuum of 'arousal.' Then there comes a tipping point between peak excitement and what we think of as stress.

The theory is that there is a state where we are fine, living in a state of concentration and focus, which does have elevated heart rate, heightened brain activity, and slightly elevated hormone levels. Going over the edge is when we very suddenly feel we are no longer capable of managing what's in front of us. The 'challenge' that we were okay dealing with has turned into a 'threat' which we don't believe we can handle, or we sense that the perceived danger is overwhelming. Scientists refer to the state where we're okay as 'eustress,' and the state where we aren't as 'distress.'

Human bodies are the result of millions of years of evolutionary adaptation that have allowed us to survive. The physiological response to distress is the same as if we were being chased by a lion. The body reacts with a release of adrenaline related hormones and a diversion of blood away from the brain and stomach towards our muscles. This leaves us feeling queasy, lightheaded, and not able to think as clearly. Under threat, our mental capacities are compromised in favor of sending blood and energy to our muscles.

These responses to distress are useful and appropriate when our physical survival is threatened. They aren't helpful when we are facing modern, everyday threats whether they are to our career, relationships, reputation, finances, or whatever. When feeling overwhelmed by the demands of the job, of family life, or keeping up to date with news, social media, and changes in society, our body responds by flooding us with powerful chemicals and sending blood to our muscles.

One of the other problems with our stress response when we feel overwhelmed, is that many today are feeling overwhelmed all of the time. I used to like putting together to-do lists so that I could get that little dopamine rush by crossing things off. Now I find it hard to put the list together because there is too much on it; I know I will fail to do everything I 'have' to do, and that is stressful. Better to flail away without facing up to the impossible. For many of us, we are trying to be successful at our jobs to get ahead, we are trying to be healthy, exercise, eat right, we are trying to find or maintain our relationships with all of the complexity that entails, we are trying to stay in touch with friends, trying to keep up on social media, trying to stay on top of news, trying to read a book once in a while, trying to contribute, and trying to do something fun occasionally. It doesn't seem possible.

The distress response was designed to get us ready on the rare occasions we were actually physically threatened, which even a long, long time ago wouldn't have been all day, every day. Wild animals don't get the stress-related diseases we get because they only get 'stressed' for short periods of time. They don't live under a continual, chronic distress response, and our bodies aren't designed to live that way either. The links between chronic stress levels as measured by hormone levels such as cortisol and chronic health issues such as heart disease and cancer are well documented. Living under continual, chronic distress is killing us.

So stress, or at least living with a continual distress response is unhealthy. No rocket science there. But what does meditation do to alleviate that?

What Happened When a Molecular Biologist Went to the Monastery

In the late 1970s, a molecular biologist at the University of Massachusetts Medical Center went to an old Catholic monastery in Barre, Massachusetts that had been converted into a Buddhist meditation retreat center. While there, he had the insight that this meditation thing could be really good for the many people in his hospital who were suffering. He went back to the hospital and started teaching some meditation practices without the Buddhism part. His name was Jon Kabat-Zinn, and the program he established is today known as the Mindfulness Based Stress Reduction program (MBSR).

MBSR lasts eight weeks and is a fairly intensive program requiring participants to commit to doing about forty-five minutes of practice a day, six days a week, for the duration. Practice varies between basic yoga and different types of awareness meditation.

Thanks to Kabat-Zinn, tens of thousands of people have now gone through a repeating program such that scientists have been able to study the effects since 1979. The early research into this program showed such promise that it caused scientific interest in meditation to increase almost exponentially over the last thirty years. The findings suggest that MBSR works. It dramatically reduces the stress response in its participants, along with numerous other benefits such as improved immune responses, lower blood pressure, better sense of well-being, and decreased suffering from chronic pain.

Kabat-Zinn has pointed out the irony that when people are asked several weeks after doing his program what part of it had the most effect, they tend to say the breathing. As he says, this seems odd since they were clearly breathing their whole life before they came to the program. But they hadn't been doing so with as much awareness. They possibly hadn't been doing it properly either, and he gets them breathing into their bellies, formally known as diaphragmatic breathing or abdominal breathing. That alone, completely independent of any meditation, can stimulate a relaxation response in the body. So if you do nothing else – do that. Take five, slow, deep breaths into your belly and notice the difference.

That's not meditation. But it is what might be referred to as mindful breathing. Being conscious of your breathing is a first step towards meditation.

It is tempting to explain what else in the meditation program leads to relaxation, but any explanation is a reduction. I can give you some theory as to why it works, but it is not the whole story. To some extent, you just have to do it, and you will find out for yourself that while my, or anyone else's explanation may make sense and may be accurate, there is more to the experience.

One way in which meditation helps with stress was illustrated in the Killingsworth and Gilbert study at Harvard. When we are thinking, thinking, thinking, or at least ruminating about our lives, we are not terribly happy. Whatever the pressures on our lives at any given moment, thinking constantly about how stressed we are and how difficult it all is, makes the problem worse. Meditating, even for a few minutes can interrupt that pattern while we put our attention somewhere else.

Another aspect is what I think of as the fish tank syndrome. If you have a fish tank, where the water is nice and still, it looks clear. But if you stir the water around it gets very cloudy, very quickly. If you let the water sit for a while, the big particles fall back to the bottom, and the water is clear again. When we are relentlessly thinking, and particularly when under pressure, we are stirring everything around in our minds and cannot see a way through. Meditation puts that on hold, and you can start to see what's what. Your thoughts still happen, but they settle at least somewhat, and you can start to tell one from another. You get some clarity. It doesn't change the situation, but it can completely change how you see the situation.

Stress Is About the Perception of Reality, Not Reality Itself

One key aspect of stress is the fact that it is not the nature of the situation that causes us stress. It is not whether a situation is possible or not, or whether it is likely or not. It is whether we *perceive* it to be possible or likely, or not. That is incredibly important and helpful to realize. It may have saved my life.

About ten years ago I found myself at the top of a mast in the middle of the night somewhere in the Atlantic Ocean during a storm. I was attached on a rope and being hoisted up to go and retrieve the top part of a sail that had ripped apart in the wind. The boat was rocking from side to side on the waves, so there was an extra rope to hold me close to the mast.

Unfortunately, when I was about fifty-five feet up, and above the lights so that no one below could see me, the boat hit a wave particularly hard. I lost the rope holding me close to the mast and I started swinging. No one could see me, and the wind was too loud for anyone to hear me yell. I had no control over the swing and kept bashing into the mast at high speed.

There was a moment when I realized I could die here if I hit my head, or broke something badly and was unable to help myself up or down. There was a moment of fear, but then there was also a moment of awareness of the fear. I knew that worrying about my situation was unhelpful. I had taught enough classes about stress to know that if I started to worry about dying, I could quickly send myself over the edge into "distress." If that happened, I was going to lose my ability to perform at my best.

In that moment, it was true that I might die there, but to have the best chance of not dying I had to avoid thinking about that and stay calm. The reality of the situation was irrelevant. I needed to focus on what I could do, and block out what might happen. After what seemed like forever, I got lucky, and one of the swings landed me on the main sail, which cushioned the blow, and I was able to reach over, grab the mast, reattach myself and finish the job with only a few bruises.

Once you can recognize that your stress is the result of your perception of your situation, you can change the stress. You can't change the situation with that awareness, but changing your perception will decrease your reaction to the situation. This will make you more effective. Decreasing the stress is also the healthier option.

Awareness meditation, for example focusing on your breathing, trains you in putting your focus somewhere, and then in noticing when your focus is not where you want it, and then in putting it back to where you want it. Under stress, the first thing you need to notice is that you are stressed. Then you need to notice what it is about your situation that is causing you stress. Your situation is your situation. It may be terrible. But it is your reaction to the situation that is causing the feeling of stress. Being in "distress" is unhelpful, so what can you do, where can you put your focus so that you won't feel so stressed? Putting your focus on what you can do, rather than what you can't do reduces the stress response. Meditation trains you in how to do that.

Meditation Makes You Younger

Despite the fact that the *New York Times* seems to have an almost daily article about how meditation and mindfulness are good for you, often citing some new study, there is still a lot of resistance to scientific research that appears to validate the benefits of meditation. One of the controversial pieces of research was done by Nobel prize winning geneticist, Elizabeth Blackburn with Elissa Epel, which suggested that meditation makes you younger.

I'm deliberately over-simplifying the research. In part, this is because I have noticed that people really pay attention at this point of a meditation class when I suggest that meditation may have rejuvenating properties. So if it piques your interest, it is what I'm trying to do. But it also shows how research like Blackburn and Epel's becomes controversial when people, like me, take some scientific findings and extrapolate way beyond what the data is suggesting. Nevertheless, stick with me, because their research is important and the findings are amazing.

Every strand of your DNA comes with a small protective cap on the end, called its telomere. Over time as the DNA replicates, this protective cap gets smaller and smaller until it no longer does its job as well, and the DNA is not properly protected. This can cause the DNA to end up replicating poorly, which in turn can lead to aging and disease. As you get older, your body parts literally don't work as well as they used to.

Blackburn was an expert in telomeres and was asked by Epel to take part in a study of women who were living under extreme stress. They were mothers looking after their chronically ill or disabled children.

One of the things they measured was the amount of the chemical telomerase in the bloodstream of the mothers. Telomerase is a hormone that appears to help in the health of the telomeres. The amount of telomerase decreases as we get older, which may be why the telomeres start to degrade. The researchers observed that the amount of telomerase in these women was seriously low. It was as if the women were far older than they really were. Some of the women were then invited to take part in a meditation and stress reduction program to see what the effect was. The amount of the telomerase in the women who took the course was significantly higher after the course than it had been before they meditated.

Many of my meditation colleagues feel as though they can tell how your meditation practice is going just by looking at you. I guess I feel the same way. There's a look that seems to be there, a clarity in the eyes, a positivity, an energy, a posture that's there when someone is practicing regularly, and an absence when you suspect that they have fallen off in their practice. This is completely unscientific and may be rubbish, but it is a widely held belief in the world of meditation that practitioners look younger than their age. There are exceptions of course, but there are many examples for whom it seems to apply. The Dalai Lama doesn't look in his eighties, Thich Nhat Hanh and Sharon Salzberg also seem completely immune to aging. We could put that down to genetics for sure, or good skin care perhaps. Some researchers have suggested that the youthful look of elderly monks is more to do with their staying out of the sun and being indoors to meditate than the actual meditation itself. Yet the research of Blackburn and Epel certainly made many of us in the meditation community wonder if she was providing some scientific support for what we believed about aging and practice.

If there is something to Blackburn's research, it seems likely that it isn't the meditation itself that is causing telomerase concentrations to increase. It is more likely that meditation is causing the body's distress response to soften. And the softening of the distress response could be the cause of higher amounts of telomerase. On that basis, it could be that people that meditate regularly and have done so for many years are simply living with less 'distress' response than the average person. This may, in turn, be what gives people that glint in their eye, merely in comparison to others who are living under more stress. Regardless – meditate! It might not make you younger – but decreasing your stress response could make you age less quickly.

Decreasing your stress response is likely going to lower your chances of cancer, heart disease, anxiety, and other ailments. It won't make you live forever. The Buddha died. It won't mean you won't get cancer, heart disease, or other problems. Many people who meditate get those diseases. But today's medical advice would suggest it lowers your chances of getting stress-related diseases.

CHAPTER SIX

At Work

I studied Theology and Religious Studies at university, which is not the obvious choice for someone looking to develop a corporate career or make lots of money. It is, however, a course of study that can get you interested in different spiritual practices, which might lead you to join a meditation group at some point. This happened to me, and my meditation practice then resulted in me becoming a management consultant on Wall Street.

In the summer of 1992, I found myself in San Francisco with some time to kill. I had graduated from university the previous year, and my career was headed towards doing something "worthwhile" in overseas aid or public policy. I was spending the summer in California before heading back to London where I had an offer to do a post-graduate degree in International Relations. Until this point of the year, I'd been working on that year's U.S. presidential campaign which had involved traveling all over the country, working a lot more than a hundred hours a week, surviving mostly on donuts, coffee, and no sleep. My candidate had done well in the primaries but ended up second, and the campaign was ending. I was exhausted in every way possible, physically, mentally, emotionally, and spiritually. By chance, I saw an advertisement for free meditation classes at the Unitarian Church on Geary Street in San Francisco. I'd done some meditation at university and thought that this might be exactly what I needed. Free was very attractive since I had very little money, but a little suspicious – what was the catch? Was there going to be an upsell, was this a cult?

I walked into class and was immediately put off. The person teaching the class was wearing a suit and tie which is not the go-to uniform of spiritual types who teach meditation, but I stuck around to at least do some practice. After a while, I could tell the guy did seem to know what he was talking about, and then finally it was time to meditate. It might have been the way in which he taught it, it might have been the technique or the setting in the church, but the meditation was incredible.

There was a stillness, an awareness, a peace, and all with energy and a sense of joy that I'd never experienced in meditation before. The truth is that meditation is often work, you sit and focus. You get distracted, you refocus. But sometimes there is an amazing experience to be discovered. This was one of those times. I went up to the guy at the end and asked when he was teaching again.

Fairly soon I found myself part of a small meditation community studying under his teacher. It was an intense group that took meditation very seriously and practiced various techniques from different traditions. The teacher was inspiring, funny, irreverent, and creative. He was also surprisingly practical for a meditation instructor. One of the themes of his teaching was for us to use our jobs as a tool for our practice, and also that we could use our meditation to leverage our careers.

Meditation requires focus and concentration as you develop your awareness of each moment as it unfolds. As it was explained to us, we could choose to train our minds only when we were meditating, sitting in a chair or on a cushion. Or we could enhance that to train our minds via everything we did. Whether we were doing laundry, sweeping floors, working in McDonald's, or as a doctor in a hospital, we had the opportunity in each and every second to watch our minds and to try to stay present to what we were doing in that moment.

Using meditation for career was simply the flip side of that. Employers never have enough great employees. They may have many employees, but good ones are always in short supply. If you are meditating every day, if you are working on your focus and concentration, if you are not living all of your day inside your head, behind your eyes and looking in, but spending some of the time looking out, aware of your inner world and also of the outer world, then you would be one of the good ones.

You would be different from almost everyone else out there. It doesn't make you a better person, it's merely a choice you've made about how to take control of your mind, but it will make you a better employee. Employers are desperate for people who are trying to be continually focused on what they are doing. People that meditate are more aware of their internal world, their feelings, and have better emotional regulation. They are also aware of what is going on around them and are more sensitive to other people. So long as you have the technical skills for a job, most of which can be learned with study, you will find yourself a valued asset inside a company.

The teacher took that to the next level by pointing out that unless we were going off to a monastery to practice, we were going to need money. Money worries seemed to be one of the things that caused a lot of misery in our society, so he suggested we find the simplest way to leverage the skills of meditation to make more money than we needed. Then the money problem would be solved, and we could get on with our meditation practice, go on retreats whenever we felt like it, and live wherever we wanted.

The teaching was simple. Since ultimately it didn't really matter to us what we did, we might as well pick a field that paid well – any job could act as a vehicle for training the mind. Train up so that you know everything you need to know to do the job. Meditate. That is, meditate and do the job in a way that used the meditation and simultaneously enhanced the meditation practice. Become one of the best people at that job. Not necessarily the most knowledgeable, but be competent enough technically as well as self-aware, diligent, honest, hard working, focused, and emotionally resilient. Who wouldn't want to hire someone like that?

For most of us, it took a couple of years to train up in whatever field we were in, and eventually many of us ended up as consultants. As a consultant, you take on a certain amount of risk. A company can hire and fire you whenever they feel like it without needing a reason. You get no benefits. You get no paid vacation. But you get paid a premium for taking this risk, and for us the risk was minimal. Once companies hired us as consultants, they very rarely wanted to let us go and paid premium rates to keep us.

So despite having a degree in Theology and Religious Studies, I eventually found myself working as a highly paid consultant on Wall Street. I was surprised that it worked out. I had heard all the reasons I've given you about why meditation works for your career but remained as skeptical as you may be having just read it. I was lucky that I got to find out for myself that it is true and saw hundreds of people in that meditation community do the same.

In the event that you remain doubtful about the amorphous nature of 'improving awareness, emotional regulation, focus, and concentration' as tools for your career, there are also some extremely concrete ways a meditation practice gives you an edge in the corporate world.

Creativity

I used to teach meditation at an acting school in New York City. The class was not confined to people in the school, and we would get friends of actors, friends of friends, musicians, and people walking in off the street. Most of the time I didn't know what someone's background was, or their reasons for coming to class.

One day someone asked the question, "What is the point of meditation?" I turned it back to the audience. I asked them what they were getting out of the class. A few people spoke about focus. Someone talked about improving their ability to connect to their acting partner. Others talked about it helping them manage nerves and stage fright. Finally, one woman hadn't spoken, so I asked her directly.

"I don't know" she said, "but I'm writing a children's book. At the end of every class, I always know what the next chapter's going to be about."

I am going to argue here that meditation can help you with creativity, but creativity and meditation is a complicated topic. Many meditators report similar experiences to the woman in my class. Yet scientific research into the link between creativity and meditation has been inconclusive. Some research shows upticks in creativity. Other research has not found any correlation.

Creativity: The Censor

Regardless of what science has found so far, there are a couple of concrete ways in which meditation helps creativity by *allowing* you to be more creative. Julia Cameron is a creativity coach and author of *The Artist's Way*. In her book she argues that everyone is creative, the challenge is merely in learning how to uncover your already existing talent. She explains that one of the biggest reasons you aren't as creative as you could be is because you listen to the conversation you have with yourself that says you aren't creative, or that you shouldn't be creative. She personifies this conversation as being with a character in your head, which she refers to as The Censor. This is the voice that is trying to protect you from shame and embarrassment, so it stops you from taking risks and exploring possibilities. The reason some people are more prolific creatively than others, is simply because they are able to either silence The Censor or have learned techniques for not listening to it.

I had a Censor in my head that tried to discourage me from writing this book in the first place, and is still working away while I'm writing it. It is the voice that says, "who are you to write a book about meditation," "you can't write," "it's boring," "it's self-indulgent," "how will you feel if everyone laughs at your failure," "your friends might suddenly understand who you really are and no longer like you," "no one will buy it," "those that do buy it won't read it," "there are plenty of books on meditation already, no one needs yours."

Your Censor may say different things, but everyone has one, and they exert too much influence on our willingness to explore and take risks. To make something new is always about risk; whether you are writing a book, painting, singing, decorating your house, acting, or even playing sports and trying a new way of doing something. If we do it the safe way, we will not be laughed at, but we will live in a box without ever experiencing the thrill of creating something new and original. Creativity requires us to be able to recognize that voice in our head for what it is, and to then find ways of quieting it down, or of not paying attention.

Meditation helps do this. Sometimes The Censor gets the better of me for a while; I have still got paralyzed at times while writing this book. But meditation trains us to see our thoughts for what they are, just thoughts, not truth. We develop the ability to step back for a moment and see where we are focused. Are we focused on being original, being ourselves, and taking risks, or are we focused on being safe and not living up to our creative potential?

Creativity: Separating Generation from Evaluation

When I worked for a psychology training company, we had another way of presenting creativity. We taught people to see creativity as a process with multiple stages. One stage is where we generate ideas. There is a separate stage, which is the evaluation of the ideas. As soon as we see an idea, most of us immediately form an opinion as to whether the idea is any good or not. However, if you are evaluating at the same time as you are generating ideas, you will fail to generate many ideas. The idea generation stage requires freedom from criticism so that several, maybe even hundreds or thousands of possibilities are imagined before being evaluated.

There is a saying attributed to Thomas Edison that if you want a good idea, start with ten thousand. However, you can't get to ten thousand if every time you have an idea you look at it and say – that's rubbish. Most of the ideas you will come up with are rubbish, of course, but without many, many bad ideas, you won't give yourself the freedom to find a good one.

This seems like useful information. Except it's not. It may be interesting knowledge to understand why generation and evaluation need to separate. It is interesting, but it is insufficient without the mental training to be able to separate them in your mind. The training that meditation offers is the training to notice what your mind is thinking, and the ability to redirect it so that you are focused in the direction you want to be focused. Whether it is noticing The Censor, or noticing your evaluating mind, it is this awareness of your own thoughts that allows you to be creative. Meditation offers the training to create that awareness.

The Soft Skills Myth

I consider myself extremely lucky that I like learning. I enjoy finding things out, developing new skills, trying things I've never done before. As a result, I sign up for all sorts of classes, and during my career, I have been to hundreds of development sessions. Some were useful. Some were a complete waste of time.

If you divide learning and development classes into two types, there are the technical classes and the soft skills classes. Technical being the classes where you learn the detail of how to do a job, whether it is computer programming, accounting, law, engineering, medicine, teaching, project management, or whatever. These are the well-defined things you need to know to do a job. However, technical skills are usually only half of what makes someone effective. Anything significant in complexity needs more than one person to do it, and then you run into the difficulty of people trying to deal with people. As a result, there are books, courses, and companies selling training in how to get people to improve their interactions with other people. It is this group of classes that I want to challenge and suggest that while these learning and development intentions are good, they are almost all a complete waste of time and money. I know because I not only took a lot of those classes, I've taught many of them.

I was consulting as a project manager at a European bank in London, and everyone on the team had to go to a class on how to implement change in organizations. This had become a specialty of mine, and I didn't want to waste my time. I was cocky enough to think I wouldn't learn anything, but it was mandatory, so I went. The class shocked me and ended up changing the direction of my career.

The class was dynamic, interactive, engaging, and helped me see my job in a whole new way. The information I got was useful, but what really impressed me was the way it was taught. I was sufficiently intrigued that I did some more research into this company that had such a different approach to training. They specialized in 'bite sized' 90-minute sessions that aimed to introduce various aspects of psychology and help people be more effective in the workplace as well as in their personal lives. I was hooked, and when they published a book, I bought a copy for my team. We got together once a week to discuss the next chapter. The book was interesting and I was getting bored with what I was doing, so I applied for a job with the training company.

They didn't know what to make of me since I had no experience as a corporate trainer. But they sent me about twenty psychology books to study and accepted me for their one-week in-house course on how to deliver their content their way. Somehow I passed and became a part-time trainer for them. I still was able to work as a consultant at investment banks, but every so often I would get a call to see if I wanted to teach a course for a client on a particular date. It could be about influence, negotiation, motivation, conflict management, creativity, or another of the hundred or so subjects they offered. The client might have been an oil company, or a pharmaceutical firm, an investment bank or in retail, and seeing inside so many different organizations and industries was fascinating. If I accepted, they would provide me with the course details which would enable me to learn about the subject. I would then show up somewhere in the world on a particular date to deliver the session.

The material was incredible. The latest findings from various pieces of psychological research were packaged in practical ways for people to learn useful tricks for being more effective. I loved doing it, and the clients loved the courses. As I got more competent at delivery, the training company would trust me with more and more work until I ended up doing it more or less full time.

I remember a particularly nice moment when I had been giving a session about managing different personality types, and someone came up to me afterwards to thank me and explained with tears in his eyes that this was going to change his life. He had been thinking for years that the problems he was having with his staff were because of them, but he now realized that it wasn't them at all, it was him.

I sincerely hope it helped him. It might have. I doubt it did though. The reason being that it wasn't helping me. I was learning huge amounts of information about the psychology of people, about how to be more effective, about how to interact better, and the difference in my life was minimal. It wasn't that it was completely useless, but if this knowledge helped, then the other trainers at the company and I would have been the most skillful operators on the planet. We knew how to manage every kind of person and how to recognize behavior types. We knew motivational modalities, how to think more positively, how to be more creative, to negotiate, to influence and persuade people. But the truth was that this knowledge was close to useless. We were good trainers which is why we were doing this job. We had better than average communication skills, had the ability to hold attention, transfer knowledge clearly, and do so in an engaging manner. Yet despite all the knowledge we had acquired from teaching we were only marginally more effective than when we started teaching. Most of us remained very normal people struggling like everyone else with our human limitations.

The problem is that psychology does a great job of finding out how people behave, and why people behave the way they do. It can predict with great accuracy what percentage of people will react a certain way to certain events. So I know that if for example, the waitress at my diner leaves a mint with the check, my tip is likely to be, on average, 15% more than if she didn't leave the mint. When someone asks me to do something and gives me a reason starting with the word 'because,' I am 50% more likely to agree than if they didn't give me a reason. Yet I am still a human. I can see my behavior, I can understand what I'm doing, and why I'm doing it, but the knowledge alone does not change my behavior.

In one class I would teach people many different influencing tactics, and then explain how the real skill of influence is to combine different tactics into an influencing strategy. When people learned this, they were excited to get information they didn't have before. They would walk out of the session and believe that they now knew how to be more effective at getting people to do what they wanted. And they did. They did know how. But that knowledge won't help them. It won't change how they try to influence and persuade people.

One reason that new knowledge is not going to help is that people already have strongly established habits of doing what they do the way they do it. Today, when they are trying to influence someone, they might use logic as their tactic ("because meditation gives you clarity") or perhaps they will use third party references ("Rupert Murdoch, Oprah Winfrey, and the Golden State Warriors meditate"). They might use inspiration as their tactic ("picture yourself when you are at your happiest. Now imagine yourself two years from now being that happy twice as often as you are today"), or they might use authoritative research ("Dr. Sara Lazar's research at Harvard University suggests meditation changes your brain structure and makes you happier"). But whichever tactics they have always relied on will be the tactics they continue to rely on. Habits are powerful and extremely difficult to change.

The second reason is that in order for people to be able to implement the knowledge they need an incredible degree of self-awareness at all times. They need to be able to see what they are doing when they are doing it. But most of us operate on automatic pilot, most of the time. Our automatic pilot is our series of learned behaviors that we know work in the majority of situations we deal with on a daily basis. Our automatic pilot works well enough to have got us to wherever we are in life. We can operate reasonably successfully without constantly checking in to see what we are doing, why we are doing it, or asking ourselves if this is the time to implement the knowledge we learned at that seminar on influence. Self-awareness is the missing piece. Without it, all the soft skills knowledge and psychological findings are useless.

If you start meditating, you will not immediately become more self-aware. Self-awareness develops slowly. You will slowly become more aware of your thought patterns. You will slowly develop more awareness of your feelings as you are having them. You will gradually develop more awareness of your reactions to things as they occur. As you develop these things, you will then be able to see yourself acting in the moment as it happens, and then be able to decide whether your default behavior is the one you want, or if you want to try something else.

Regular meditation is the process to get you this ability. Even now, after more than thirty years of meditating, I still operate on automatic pilot a lot of the time. But the training of meditation does increase your ability to be self-aware. Not all the time, but at least when you decide you want to be self-aware. And however slow meditation may be in developing this skill, it remains by far the best training (if not the only training) that exists to get you there. You cannot simply become more self-aware because you want to be, or because you read that it's good for you. It takes work. Meditation is that work.

Corporate human resource departments tend to be staffed by well-meaning people who have a sincere interest in helping people. But they have a difficult job trying to balance conflicting pressures inside an organization. The company wants to develop its staff and make them more productive, and it wants to have high performing, healthy and mostly happy employees. But it wants to achieve that at the most efficient price point.

Corporations also have to manage the desires and expectations of employees to get career advancement and training. Employees are usually promised they will have access to Learning and Development courses when they are hired. HR needs to deliver on those promises within the constraints of budget and in terms of what the person can realistically achieve. Soft skills training could really help people, and people want to get better at this stuff, but without training in self-awareness or mindfulness, which really means meditation training, none of the soft skills training they offer is going to make any difference.

Self-awareness is the foundational skill that needs to be taught before any of the other useful stuff has a chance of helping.

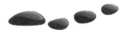

Meetings

Imagine a corporate meeting. There are eight people sitting around a conference table, some with pens and notebooks, some with laptops open. A variety of drink containers from plastic water bottles to coffee cups are arrayed. There is a conference phone in the middle of the table, and half dozen people are dialed in from remote locations. Someone is presenting a status update. Everyone is paying attention.

Except that is not what is happening. The research from the Harvard study by Killingsworth and Gilbert suggests that on average people are distracted 47% of the time. That means that on average, only 53% of people will be paying attention at any given moment. However, the

Harvard numbers are skewed high by high-focus activities such as sex where people are only distracted about 15% of the time. When I asked a colleague from the meditation community (who is now a Managing Director at a top Wall Street investment bank) if 50% sounded reasonable, she thought that was "very high." Her guess was that maybe, on a good day, people are paying attention 30-40% of the time.

Unless you are the person who organized the meeting, most of the other people don't want to be there. This meeting does not help them. They have other priorities, other problems to solve, other things they would rather be doing. They walk in with a huge number of pressures. Their to-do list is already impossible, their inbox is insane, the problems they are trying to solve need their full attention, and that is only the work aspects of their life. Their personal life is also walking into the room with them, as they wonder about trying to keep their relationship alive, their fitness, diet, health, their kids, and maybe they also dream about doing something fun one day to justify why they do this job in the first place.

When you sit down to meditate and intend to try to keep your mind focused in a particular direction, such as on your breathing, you discover it is very difficult to keep it there. The mind, all on its own, wants to run all over the place and think about other things. That happens when you are trying to stay focused. When people are sitting in a meeting that they would rather not be in, the chances of them staying focused are a lot smaller than average.

Sometimes this is obvious. Some people don't hesitate before picking up their phone to check every time it vibrates and then type off a reply. Somebody has usually dialed into the meeting who never learned how to mute their phone, and everyone can hear them on their keyboard, probably working through their email. A few people are polite and keep looking each other in the eye, appearing to listen. Even these people are probably not paying attention and instead are working out in their mind how they are going to get everything done that they need to do.

If you stop to think about this for a second, the consequences are not subtle. Companies try to keep everyone aligned and working toward common goals, and meetings are often ways in which everyone is supposed to be staying in touch with what everyone else is doing. But at best only fifty percent of anything being said is being absorbed and likely a lot less. This is easy to demonstrate by going to a presentation and asking people afterwards to write down what they think were the main points. Everyone will have different answers. This explains a large part of the dysfunction companies have in keeping everyone moving in the same direction.

The people that spend the most time in meetings are usually the most senior and highest paid. At least half that money is completely wasted since they aren't paying attention. That alone is a big number. Then there's the whole aspect of the at least 50% that everyone is missing in these meetings that leads to confusion, misdirection and a series of other problems. This, in turn, wastes more time and resources to fix those problems. A meeting that was supposed to result in people moving in the same direction ends up causing people to go in different directions because they were paying attention to different parts.

Meditation

Meditation helps us realize how distractible our minds are. Once you start from this knowledge, you realize that people are not 'present' a lot of the time. This can change how you approach meetings. If you recognize that everyone is walking into a room with dozens of different pressures and problems on their mind it can change the way you start. Some companies that are adopting more 'mindful work' approaches start meetings with a 'purposeful pause.' Personally, I think that sounds like someone should bring out the patchouli oil, light an incense candle and chime some bells, but I acknowledge that the point of the pause makes sense. It acts as a reset button, to try to get people to be aware of what they are carrying in their minds as they come into the meeting, and for the next few minutes, at least, to try to get them to focus, to be present, and to pay attention.

Curiosity

If you accept that everyone's minds are all over the place, and you want to hold their attention, use curiosity.

One of the most common communication tools in large organizations is the PowerPoint presentation. People agonize over making perfect slides that get printed out into a 'deck,' and are handed out at the beginning of a meeting. There is a theory that the deck should substitute for a document, and that someone should be able to review the deck at a future point in time and know what happened in the meeting. Really? If you don't have time to pay attention in the meeting in the first place, you're not going to have time to go back and review it later.

The alternative? Use PowerPoint as it was intended, as a presentation aid. If you need a supporting document with the detail, do that. It is so much easier than trying to work out what sized font you need in order to get all the words on a slide. In a document, you can use as many words as you need to make your point. Use the slides instead to make people curious about what you're about to say. Put up images instead of words. Words either a) get them reading your slide which means they're not paying attention to what you're saying, or more likely, b) send everyone straight to sleep.

Using images is a simple but powerful presentation trick where you create intrigue. You're going to be talking about the budget, but you put up a slide of a five-year-old playing on a beach. You now have their attention. They are curious. They have no idea why you have put up a slide with a kid with a bucket and spade. Their curious mind wants to know. You now have the opportunity to make the point you need to make about the budget. Ideally, you somehow bring it back to the sand in the bucket, maybe making some kind of point about the sand in the bucket versus sand on the beach, or whatever. It doesn't even need to be very clever; you only need to get people to give you a few minutes of attention. Do this, and you're ahead of nearly every other person presenting.

Awareness of the Listener

The knowledge that people are paying attention at best half the time can also change how you talk. I'm sure you can recall presentations where it is clear that the only person the presenter is talking to is the presenter. They have long since lost the audience, and everyone is waiting for them to finish. In the meantime, the audience is daydreaming or thinking about what they need to do as soon as the presentation is over.

When you are aware of how difficult it is to hold focus, you will then pay close attention to whether you still have the audience's focus, or whether you have lost it. This is another of the simple, and yet powerful presentation tricks – to pay attention to your audience, to know that you are likely to lose them at some point (even with using curiosity) and that when you have lost your audience, you stop. You don't necessarily stop the presentation, but pause. Pause for a slightly uncomfortably long time. Provided people are not fully asleep they will suddenly be interrupted from whatever mental path they were going down and look at you. If they were truly lost in thought, they are now wondering what you just said. They may even worry that you asked them a question while they weren't paying attention. For a few seconds at least, you will once again have everyone's attention.

I've never met anybody that loved meetings. Some are useful. Some are well run and efficient. Many are a waste of everyone's time. Some are critical, and for big problems, you need to get specific individuals together at the same time to go through ideas and proposals. But if you get a reputation for running bad meetings, people won't show up to the ones you organize, and you won't be able to get done what you need to get done. If you run useful, short, focused meetings that hold people's attention, they still won't want to come, but they'll recognize that it won't be a complete waste of time and are more likely to come if they can.

If you want to run good meetings, get clear about the purpose of the meeting, have an agenda, stick to it, and meditate. I don't mean that you should meditate during the meeting, but a big part of the quality of the meeting depends on the clarity of the chairperson. If you walk in, and the chair exudes a sense of certainty about what they are trying to achieve in this meeting, you have at least a sense at the beginning that this isn't going to be a complete waste of time. The meeting might even be over before the allotted hour is up, and you can then get on with some of the other things you need to be doing. If, however, you walk in and the chair is not focused, there is no clear sense of purpose or agenda, you immediately know this is a waste of time, and you start putting your mind somewhere that it might be more usefully engaged. Meditation gives you clarity. You sit, you observe your mind, you get to see what's coming into it, and where it's going. You are training yourself to distinguish between your focus and your distractions. When you walk into a meeting, whether you know it or not, other people will pick up whether you are clear, or foggy. That, in turn, will help you for those first few minutes at least, to keep people on your side.

More Than Relaxation

Many senior executives meditate. Steve Jobs may have been one of the most famous that found it helpful but the list is long. It is likely that it helps them stay calm under pressure, but for many of these people, the attraction of meditation isn't about managing stress. Most of them were good at managing stress before they meditated, which is why they rose through the ranks in the first place. What they have discovered is that meditation is good for so much more than stress management. It improves focus and helps clear the thinking. It helps you manage yourself, and other people better. It can unleash your creativity, improve communications, make you self-aware, and more.

CHAPTER SEVEN

How to Meditate

On one level meditation is very simple.

You breathe in, you breathe out.

Try to hold your attention on the breathing.

When you get distracted, bring your attention back to the breathing.

Do this over and over.

Practice this for twelve minutes a day.

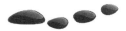

If you do this every day, you will notice the difference very quickly, and the benefits build over time.

That said, there are hundreds and maybe thousands of different techniques. Here I'm going to outline a few more to get you started, but check out RealWorldMeditation.org where there are more techniques, guided meditations, and a 12 Week Introduction to Meditation Course to help you establish a practice.

Awareness Meditation – *The Breath*

Take a breath, in and out.

That's it. More or less.

Now, get a timer. Your phone or watch is fine. Set it for three minutes.

This time, breathe normally, trying to hold your attention on your breathing. When you notice your attention has gone off the breath and you're thinking about something else, just gently return your attention to the breath.

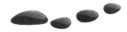

People think of meditation as hard because after the first couple of breaths it is hard to hold the attention on the breathing. That isn't the point though. You are developing your awareness, your awareness of the breath, and your awareness of your own thoughts. You are also developing your ability to move your focus from one thing to another, in this case from your thoughts back to observing your breathing.

One of the fallacies people have about meditation is that everyone else must be finding it easier than they are. In a yoga studio, you would see that most people in the class are similar to you. They are clumsy and wobbling at least as badly as you are. If we could see inside people's minds, we would see that everyone's mind was basically the same as ours.

Sometimes the mind is more distracted than at other times, but everyone's mind is always getting pulled in different directions. It's what minds do - they wander. Other people may seem to be sitting still with their eyes closed and looking peaceful, but inside, their minds are all over the place. In yoga terms, everyone would be falling over all the time. It is important to realize this. You aren't doing meditation wrong if your mind is all over the place. In yoga, it is absolutely fine to fall over. Then you start again, pick yourself up and get back into the pose. The same is true in meditation.

Applying Your Curiosity

We'll do the same exercise as before, but this time we're going to try to apply curiosity. Breathing can seem mundane. We do it all the time. We take it for granted. It is a perfect object for us to get curious about.

As you're reading this, notice your breathing. Notice how your body expands the lungs, automatically. Get a sense of your body moving as you breathe.

Now try consciously breathing into your belly (rather than your chest), noticing as the belly expands, and then contracts. See what changes as you breathe. Notice the subtle way in which you can feel the sensations of your shirt against your skin change during the inhalation and exhalation. Try this for three breaths.

Now, see if you can notice the impulse that causes your body to take the next breath. It is very quiet, but the impulse arises when some subconscious part of you wants you to take the next breath. Equally, your body knows when it has the right amount of air, and then the body relaxes, pushing the air out again.

See if you can notice that sometimes the lungs pull in more air, sometimes less.

Observe the air as it travels in your nose or mouth, see if you notice the sensation of air as it moves over your lips, or in your nostrils.

See how far you can notice the air as it travels into your lungs. Where does the awareness of the air stop? Is it at the back of the throat, at the top of your chest, or further down? This is not a test, just a prompt to help you observe the air closely, to notice how far you sense it traveling.

If you get curious about the breath, you will be able to hold your attention there a little longer before you get distracted.

Set the timer for three minutes again, close your eyes and try the meditation again, but this time seeing what happens when you get curious about your breathing.

There is a fine line between using curiosity to stay focused and then starting to think thoughts about the breathing. When people ask about whether thinking about the breathing is okay in the meditation, I tend to reply that thinking about the breathing shows their attention is on the breathing, but it is different from holding their awareness on the breathing. It may be a better quality of thought than thinking about what happened on TV last night, but it's still thinking. There is a subtle and crucial difference between *thinking* about breathing and *being aware* of the breathing. It is a delicate line that can be fun to play with in your mind. Notice when your curiosity is working to help you *observe* the breath in detail, versus when your curiosity starts you *thinking* about your breathing.

Curiosity is useful for many aspects of meditation as well as for helping you hold focus in your real life. It also works well with the next exercise, non-judgment. When you're curious, you're just looking at what's there; you are not evaluating it as good or bad.

EXERCISE #3:
Non-Judgment

In all meditations, it is important to try not to apply judgment. Not doing something can be tricky, but nevertheless, you can notice once you have started judging things, and then see if you can let the judgment go.

One common judgment people have is about their own 'meditation ability.' If your mind gets distracted, try not to criticize yourself for that. It is what minds do. Or, if you notice you are being self-critical, see if you can let that criticism go.

Set the timer for three minutes. Try the breathing exercise again but watch out for your judgment of the meditation.

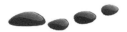

Sometimes you will be distracted constantly, and you can barely bring your attention to the breath before it is off and thinking. Sometimes you will engage a thought for a long time before realizing that you have gone down that particular track. So what? You're doing what you're supposed to be doing. You are sitting, observing, noticing when your mind has wandered and then returning the focus. Over and over.

Experienced meditators are doing exactly the same as you – they are getting distracted. The difference is they expect this. They don't fret about it. They recognize it for what it is and return the focus.

Okay, maybe this isn't completely true. Experienced meditators still judge themselves for getting distracted. I still get frustrated on days when my mind is particularly distracted. But perhaps we catch the judgment and recognize that for what it is more quickly. Either way, there is a constant training of noticing when the judging mind has kicked in.

With experience, you will also find out that although it is nice when the mind finds some stability, sometimes the biggest benefits of meditation come on the days when the mind is particularly busy.

EXERCISE #4:

The Body Scan

Focusing on the breath is powerful, classic, and simple. Not easy, but it is simple. A variation is to move the focus to your entire body, to develop your awareness of the sensations of the body.

Your body is sending you thousands of signals every second. You aren't paying attention to most of those since they aren't urgent or 'important,' but the signals are getting sent anyway. Your feet are aware of how the floor feels. If you are sitting down, you can feel the weight of your body in the seat. Your shoulders may feel heavy as the arms hang. Your skin is aware of where your clothing is touching and where it is not. Your skin and body are sensitive to temperature, and every part of your body is telling you how hot or cold they are. Most of the time they are within the range of what's acceptable, so you ignore the information, but the information is always there if you pay attention.

You can do this meditation while sitting, standing, or lying down, but however you want to do it, you will probably find it easier to do while listening to a guided version. You can find a 'Body Scan Meditation' on RealWorldMeditation.org, and there are many variations elsewhere on the internet.

If you don't have access to a guided version, read through this and get a sense of what you're doing, and then try leading yourself through it.

Take a nice deep breath in. And let it out.

Take another deep breath in and as you let it out, see if you can release any tension you're feeling.

Take another deep breath in. Let it go.

See if you can notice how your body is feeling overall.

If you're tired, anxious, annoyed, happy, relaxed, or something else, just notice what is true without judging. Try to avoid getting into a story in your mind about whether it's good or bad. Just notice what is true about how you're feeling right now.

Take your focus to your left foot and try to become aware of the big toe on your left foot. Just becoming aware of it. Seeing if you can feel it. See if you can feel the pressure of the floor, your shoe, or a sock. Are you aware if it's touching the other toe?

Now move your attention to the second toe on your left foot. If you have to wiggle it slightly to feel it, go ahead.

Your middle toe.

Fourth toe.

Your little toe.

Now become aware of the ball of your foot.

Notice if there is pressure from the floor.

Then moving along the arch of your foot towards your heel. Noticing, if you can feel where the pressure of the floor is and is not pressing into the foot.

See if you can become aware of the top of your foot.

Moving your attention towards your ankle.

Notice if there's any tension in the ankle. Any sensation. Again, without judging it. Just notice what's true.

Now become aware of the whole of your left foot, all the way from the ankle to your toes.

Now move the attention up to the calf.

Maybe you can notice the fabric of clothes on your skin. Maybe notice where it's not touching.

Moving your attention up towards the knee.

Become aware of the knee itself. This is an incredibly complex joint. They get injured a lot. Often cause us pain. Just see if you can sit in awareness of the knee without talking to yourself about it.

If you can, get curious about any sensations you're getting from your knee.

Then move the attention to the back of the top part of your leg. Noticing where it is touching anything.

Up to the hip. Aware of any pressure from the floor, or seat, and where there is no pressure.

Noticing where skin is aware of being in contact with anything.

Now move your attention along the top of the upper leg. From the knee, along the big muscle on the top. To the hip.

Now become aware of the whole of your left leg, from the hip all the way to the tips of your toes. Any individual sensations, or all the sensations at once. Notice what your leg is telling you from touch or pressure, or from aches and pains.

Now move your attention to the right foot.

To the big toe on your right foot.

Then your second toe.

Third toe. If you have to wiggle them a bit to feel them, go ahead, so you get a sensation.

Your fourth toe.

And your little toe. Become aware of any pressure from the floor. Your socks if you have them, your shoes.

Move your attention to the ball of the foot, on the bottom.

Becoming aware of the arch.

Then moving towards the heel.

Then becoming aware of the top of your foot. Moving towards your ankle. If there is any pain there, just get curious. Look at it closely. What is the nature of that pain?

Now you're aware of the whole of your right foot, from the ankle to the toes.

Then move the attention up the back of the lower leg, becoming aware of the calf.

Now move your attention up the front of the lower leg. Becoming aware of your shin.

Then moving up to your knee.

Then become aware of the bottom part of your upper leg. The big hamstring muscle. Moving your attention towards your hip.

Now notice the top of the upper part of the leg. See if you can notice where the fabric of your clothes is touching and where it is not.

Then become aware of your hip.

Finally becoming aware of the whole of your right leg, from your hip all the way to the toes. Noticing all of the sensations at once.

Then move your attention towards the lower back.

Some people say we store stress and anger here in the lower back. Just notice what's there. Without the story. Noticing if you're holding tension here. Becoming aware of it.

Move up to the middle of the back. Noticing where your back is touching anything, and where it's not.

Then moving focus all the way to the shoulders.

Now aware of the whole of your back. Noticing where there are aches and pains. Trying not to judge them. Just noticing what's true.

Now move your attention to your belly. Noticing how it expands and contracts with the breath. Noticing any feelings, any sensations.

Moving up to your chest.

The center of your chest is sometimes associated with joy, love, and balance. But sometimes we also experience sadness here. Noticing just what you feel here without dwelling on it or creating a story about it.

Now move your attention to the top of your chest all the way to where it meets your throat.

Become aware of the whole of the front of your body. Bringing your attention into present time by noticing what your body is telling you right now. It might be a loud message; it might be a soft message. Just be aware. Just noticing what's true.

Then become aware of the shoulders.

This is another place we hold a lot of tension. In conflict, we tense our shoulders. Right now we're not trying to fix it; we're just trying to notice it if it's there.

Now noticing your left arm. The top of your left arm to start with.

Down to your elbow.

Your forearm.

Your left wrist.

Your hand.

Your thumb. Forefinger. Middle finger. Fourth finger. And little finger.

Become aware of the whole of your left arm, from your shoulder all the way down to the tips of your fingers.

Now take your attention to your right shoulder.

Your right arm. Moving down to your elbow.

Your forearm.

Your wrist.

Your hand.

Your right thumb. Index finger. Middle finger. Fourth finger. And little finger. Just becoming aware of all the sensations in your right arm, from your shoulder to the tips of your fingers.

If you notice that your mind is wandering, just notice that it's wandering. Return it initially to the breath. Now bring your whole body into awareness.

Notice if you are feeling resistance, frustration, boredom, or anything else right now. See if you can stay with those feelings, and notice them. See them for what they are, feelings that are arising.

Now take your attention to your neck.

Notice the back of your neck to start with. Notice where any clothing is touching, where air is touching, maybe where your hair is touching.

Become aware of your throat.

Become aware of your jaw.

Your lower lip. Your upper lip.

Become aware of your tongue in your mouth.

Become aware of your left cheek. Your right cheek.

Notice if you're carrying any tension in your face, in your jaw.

Notice your eyes, your left eye, your right eye.

Notice if there's any pain there, again without a story or judgment, just noticing what it feels like.

And your forehead.

Notice your nose.

Your left ear.

Your right ear.

Now take a deep breath in. And let it out.

See if you can be aware of your whole body. From the top of your head to the tips of your toes. See if you can open your awareness to all the different sensations going on. Not just the loud ones, but also the subtle ones.

Take another deep breath in. And let it go.

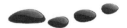

Awareness of your body's physical sensations is a powerful way of getting your attention into the present moment. Just as the breath you are having right now is only happening right now, the sensations your body is experiencing now are only happening right now.

You may experience similar feelings at other times, but the feeling you're experiencing now is only happening now. When you find yourself overwhelmed in your head, thinking too much, anxious or worried, it is a useful exercise to 'check-in' with your body, move your attention to what it is telling you right now. Immediately, even if only for a second or two, you are out of your head and in the present moment.

Awareness of Emotions

One of most common questions in our society is our daily greeting. "How are you doing?", "How's it going?", or "How are you?". Answering it honestly is surprisingly difficult for most people. "Fine," "I'm well," or "Okay" are socially acceptable but are rarely true, and are never a complete answer.

Many of us live our lives intimately familiar with what we think, what we believe, and what our opinions are. We live most of the time in the area right behind our eyes. Visually attuned to what is going on, and relentlessly turning the cogs inside our mind. But we are not as aware of our bodies, or our emotions.

I grew up in England. Emotions were generally considered unhelpful baggage that got in the way. Intellect and a stiff-upper-lip discipline were supposed to overcome them. The ideal individual was portrayed as someone very stoic in the face of any difficulty. We should rise above our emotions.

My experience living in America is that this is also an approach many have, but it is evolving. Many now respect the expression of emotion in a way that wouldn't have happened 50 or 100 years ago. Under certain circumstances, it is acceptable, or even expected that people will cry, even on live television.

One theory regarding emotions is that they emerged through the evolutionary process because they serve as messages useful for our survival. Intellect is a great resource for solving problems, learning from the past and planning for the future. Emotions are more practical for short-term survival.

In the face of a threat, it is useful to have a reaction that prepares us for action. The amygdala in the brain is the seat of our emotional life and processes information far more quickly than the intellectual part of the brain. If we are startled by a snake, the reaction is immediate and not cognitive. We don't think about it. The blood is immediately routed to our big muscles, ready for fight or flight. We get a burst of adrenaline and related hormones that heighten our senses and prepare us. We tend to freeze first, a useful survival reaction, and then are ready to move.

The etymology of emotion is linked to motion, and they are messages that prepare us to change our movement. Anger prepares us for battle. Fear, for running away or hiding. Grief and sadness turn us inward, moving us more slowly as protection to conserve energy.

I say all of this to propose that you try seeing your emotions, even the unpleasant ones, as helpful, rather than as a hindrance.

In this meditation, you are going to take a first step towards your emotional awareness and merely see if you can become aware of what you are feeling, without judging it.

Start by taking a couple of deep breaths into the belly and then allow the breathing to return to normal.

Take a few breaths holding your attention on the breathing.

Now check to see if you can notice what emotions you are feeling right now.

Notice if you are feeling sad, happy, angry, calm, anxious, joyful, or whatever you are feeling.

It may be complex.

But try to become aware of what you are feeling without judging or suppressing the feelings.

For many of us, the temptation is to repress uncomfortable feelings like sadness, anger, or anxiety. If you've never done this type of emotional awareness work, maybe you can see this exercise as an experiment in developing a different relationship with your emotions. It is not trying to say that these feelings should be 'accepted,' but it is an exercise in 'acknowledging' what is true, right now. These feelings may not be what you want to feel, but they are there. The first step is to become aware of them. Once you get better at that, then you can become more skillful at deciding what they mean, and what you want to do about them. For now, merely try to sit and notice, without judgment or conversation, what you are feeling. If you sit with the feelings for a while, they will change. See if you can notice this.

Sometimes when you do this, we can become aware of powerful, but buried feelings. Anger, sadness, hurt, resentment, grief can show up and feel horrible. This practice is not trying to be sadistic and encourages you to only sit with these as much as you can. If it is too much, back off the exercise for now and try a different meditation. However, there is much to be gained the more you can sit with them.

As I explained in the first chapter, curiosity is a tool that can help us sit with difficult feelings. As you feel unpleasant emotions, your automatic reaction might be to suppress them. The approach of meditation is to notice them, becoming aware of them, acknowledge them, and then move closer to them in your mind with curiosity. See if you can explore the feelings in detail. Where are you feeling the feeling? What texture does it have? Is it a throbbing sensation, a shooting sensation, or an all-pervasive ache? Does it change in intensity, sometimes being very strong, sometimes less strong? Is there a temperature to the feeling, for example, anger can feel hot, but fear and anxiety can seem cold. To the extent that it is unpleasant, why is it unpleasant, what is the reason you don't like it? Is the feeling energizing (anger), or depleting (sadness)?

Moving towards the unpleasant emotions with curiosity changes your relationship to the feeling. It doesn't change the emotion, but you start to see it in more detail, and it loses some of its power over you. The more you can sit with the feeling, the less you have to automatically react to it.

Open Field Awareness

Focused attention on a single thing, whether it is our breath, our bodies, or our emotions is powerful. It trains us by helping us notice when our attention has been distracted from the single object of focus.

Open field awareness meditation almost does the opposite. In open field awareness, we open our attention to everything.

You are going to sit, take a few deep breaths to settle yourself, and then relax into normal breathing. If you are a very visually oriented person, you may want to close your eyes for this exercise in order to tune in to your other senses better.

You will start with a normal breath meditation. Holding your attention on the in breath, and out breath. But then slowly start to open your other senses up to notice what they are aware of.

First, notice any physical sensations you are experiencing. Become aware of where your body is touching anything, like your feet on the floor, hands in the lap, perhaps your back against a chair, or your bottom on its seat. Notice where you are aware of clothing touching your skin and where it doesn't.

Notice what emotions you are feeling right now.

Now open yourself up to notice any sounds. Whether it is background noise like heating, air conditioning, the wind, electrical hums, or specific noises like cars, or voices. See if you can avoid naming the noises or thinking about them, and simply being aware of the information your ears are sending to your brain.

As with the breathing, it isn't so much that you try to avoid thinking, but when you notice that your mind is going down a thinking track, gently bring it back to being open to all your senses. Sitting with your awareness open to any and all sensations.

Set your timer for three minutes and try it now.

Change

You may need to set your timer for a bit longer this time. Try five minutes to start with.

This time you are going to hold yourself in open awareness as you did with the last exercise, but try to hone your attention to notice as things change within you.

See if you can notice if you get bored, or restless. Or get an itch. Or any feeling at all. If it happens, see if you can be aware of how it arose.

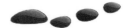

At first, you may only be able to be aware of feelings once they have arisen. You suddenly notice that you are feeling frustrated, or hungry, or something else. Or aware that you are uncomfortable and you want to move. There's nothing wrong with moving, but see if you can become aware of the change in your feelings before you react to them. Develop that space between the feeling and your response.

EXERCISE #8:
Mantra Meditation

A popular meditation alternative to awareness meditation is to sit quietly and repeat a word or phrase over and over in your mind. This is sometimes referred to as Vedic meditation or Mantra meditation. Variations of this technique can be found in most of the world's religious traditions, both in the East and the West, but does not have to be thought of, or used as a spiritual exercise.

When it comes to picking your word or phrase, some people say that the word or phrase you use matters a lot. Others say it really doesn't matter. I'm agnostic. I think it might make a difference to the quality of your experience, but I also know that using anything also works. Maybe the 'right' mantra will produce a better result, but I'm not even sure what 'better' would mean. One practitioner said he used the word "doorknob" just because it was the first thing that came into his head and he said it worked for him. I'm sure "doorknob" is fine, but I prefer some of the options found from different religions. They feel more meditation-y.

In Hindu traditions, it is common to repeat a Sanskrit word like "Om," or "Sring." In the Jewish tradition, there have been groups that repeated one or more of the different names of God, such as "Adonay," or "Elochim." Sufis within the Islamic tradition have a practice where they use some of the different names for Allah. In the Christian tradition, a phrase commonly used has been the first line of Psalm 71 – "Oh God come to my assistance, O Lord make haste to help me." In all these traditions, you repeat the mantra over and over, and the mind eventually gets quieter. Just as with the breath meditations, your mind will wander, that's what minds do, but when you notice it has gone somewhere else, you return your attention to the mantra.

I have always liked a Buddhist mantra I was taught in India, "Om Mane Padme Hum," which can be loosely translated as "happiness is within you." Om, like what people say at the end of a yoga class. Mane, approximately pronounced like money, but technically it's more like "mah-ney." Padme is Luke Skywalker's mother's name if you're a Star Wars geek, and is pronounced as "pahd-mey." Hum, as if you're humming a tune, although technically more of a "hoom" than a "hum."

You could use your own name. You could use a word like "love" or "grateful." You can pick the name of your favorite saint, Native American spirit, or whatever inspires you.

If you want your own 'special' mantra, this is the technique of one of the better-known meditation schools, Transcendental Meditation. If you take their class, they will give you a mantra specifically for you.

Or, for now, pick something. Pick anything. If it turns out you like this exercise, you have the rest of your life to experiment with different words and phrases.

Settle yourself down, set a timer for five minutes and start repeating your mantra over and over in your mind. When you notice you are distracted in your mind, gently, without judgment, return your focus to repeating the mantra.

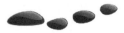

There is something very soothing about this meditation technique, and it is very popular. Transcendental Meditation's version seems to be the meditation of choice for Hollywood celebrities as well as millions of others around the world.

It is excellent as a technique for relaxation, or as an antidote to anxiety and stress. It also helps you move your attention into the present moment as opposed to wandering around the past or future inside your head. It works as a technique for noticing when the mind has been distracted and returning it to the mantra.

One of the biggest arguments in favor of this technique is that many people seem to find it 'easy,' whereas people who do awareness meditation tend to say it is 'difficult.' Perhaps this helps them stick with it better as well.

I like it, and I do use it sometimes in conjunction with other techniques. However, I think it lacks some of the training benefits that awareness meditations offer.

EXERCISE #9:

Loving Kindness Meditation

Awareness meditation and Mantra meditation both represent methods for noticing when the mind is distracted and for bringing the focus back to something. Loving Kindness Meditation is different. It is a training for awakening your compassion.

When I hear the word compassion, I worry that it is being used as a synonym for weakness or being a pushover. Alternatively, it is possible that it is also a synonym for love, whatever that might mean. If you are turned off by the term, I ask you to put that cynicism on hold and try it. This is possibly the simplest of all the meditation techniques, and yet one of the most powerful. It delivers immediate feelings of well-being, as well as delivering long-term effects in changing the way you see yourself and see others. If you've ever wondered how some people stay calm when other people are losing their heads, particularly when dealing with difficult people, screaming children, or dangerous drivers — this is the training that can get you there.

This is another meditation where it helps to listen to someone guiding you through it. You can download or stream a guided version of this from RealWorldMeditation.org. There are several other excellent versions available if you search "Loving Kindness" on the Internet.

If you don't have access to that right now, read this through and then try to guide yourself through it.

In this version of the meditation, there are five different phases, with each done for about the same amount of time. So for a ten-minute meditation, you would try to do each phase for a couple of minutes.

In the first phase, you start by picturing someone, or something very special to you. This could be a spouse, a partner, a parent, a child, a friend, or even your pet. Something where it is easy for you to picture or feel yourself sending them love. As you hold them in your mind, repeat certain phrases toward them, a little like in a mantra meditation. "May you be happy. May you be healthy. May your life be filled with joy."

In the second phase, you picture yourself and say the phrases to you. This is often the phase people find hardest, and if you experience resistance to that, notice the resistance, see if you can let go of that and open your heart to yourself. At least for this exercise.

"May I be happy. May I be healthy. May my life be filled with joy."

The third phase is to picture someone neutral in your life. It could be a colleague, a neighbor, or someone you routinely meet in your life like the person behind the counter at the post office, but it should be someone you know, and yet don't really know well enough to have positive or negative feelings toward them. See yourself sending them the same level of compassion and love, recognizing they struggle with life, just as you do. They experience sadness and loss, just as you do. They will experience grief and suffering, just as you will.

"May they be happy. May they be healthy. May their lives be filled with joy."

The fourth phase raises the level of challenge. The recommendation is to picture someone who you find a little difficult, perhaps a family member that annoys you, or a work colleague. In the beginning, it isn't recommended you try for people you feel very strongly about.

You picture this person and recognize that despite your differences, they are also someone that suffers, that experiences sadness, grief, and pain. They struggle with life, just as everyone does. See yourself sending them love and compassion, repeating the phrases over and over.

"May they be happy. May they be healthy. May their lives be filled with joy."

For the final phase, the idea is to get your heart to open completely to everyone and everything. Some people are only comfortable going with all people; some open up to all living things. Whether you choose to pick the billions of humans or the trillions of living things on the planet, you are stretching yourself to send love indiscriminately. Perhaps picture the entire planet with its billions or trillions of beings and send everyone love.

"May they be happy, may they be healthy, may their lives be filled with joy."

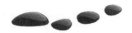

There is an epidemic of self-judgment, self-criticism and even self-hate in our society. It is one thing to be aware of our faults and strive to correct them, but it is another to relentlessly berate ourselves. This is the antidote.

People often have a hard time with the fourth phase, the difficult person in your life. May I suggest it is a tool for your training. They never need to know that you did this for them. This is not an exercise in trying to forgive them or to accept their behavior. It is for you. It is like being on the treadmill at the gym, and you are raising the incline or making it go faster. It isn't to punish yourself; it is to make you stronger. In this phase, you are working your compassion muscles harder, also to make you stronger.

Other Options: Guided, Visualizations, Combinations

Meditation is a term that covers many different techniques. Here I've shared a few of the more common ones. These are not the only types of meditation.

Guided meditations are very popular. One of the best meditation apps for smartphones at the moment is Headspace, which offers hundreds of guided meditations organized into different courses, or 'packs' for a small subscription. The Insight Timer is another excellent meditation app that is free and also has an enormous library of guided meditations. I have guided meditations on my website at RealWorldMeditation.org. Guided meditations are nice, and I use the ones on Headspace and Insight Timer from time to time. Guided meditations can help us hold our focus and can lead us to experience different states of consciousness by pointing us in certain directions. However, the emphasis of this book is on meditation as a training. A training which can help your career, your relationships, your health, happiness, and more. That isn't to say that guided meditations don't help those things, they can, but they are not as rigorous a training as meditating by yourself.

Other meditation techniques can include visualizations whereby you might picture a sandy beach, a meadow, a still lake, a river, or a certain color and do various mental exercises with that visualization in mind. Chanting out loud is a technique. There are meditation techniques that involve special breathing exercises, and many, many more. If you find techniques not mentioned here, but you like them, go ahead and keep practicing them. My only real intention in this book is to inspire you to try meditation, to establish some kind of regular practice, and to discover for yourself what is available.

If you are new to this, try a number of techniques, and find one or two, or a few that you like. Don't believe that one is the best; there is no such thing. There might just be the best one for you. And it might only be the best one for you today. Tomorrow that might change. So be open to trying new methods.

There is an argument for eventually picking a tradition, or even only one technique and sticking with it. The analogy used is that if you keep digging lots of holes for short periods of time you will never strike water, oil, or whatever it is you were digging for. It is only in continuing to dig in the same hole you will eventually get somewhere. I don't disagree with the argument except for one thing. It assumes the digging of several holes has no value in and of itself. Most people aren't looking to meditation for enlightenment, God, transcendence, mystical union, or whatever. They want more peace, more understanding, nicer relationships, less suffering, to be less yanked around by their mind and emotions, maybe to like themselves a little more. They'll take career success, improved health, and a greater sense of well-being as additional benefits. On that basis, every different type of hole you dig will help. You can learn things from every meditation, regardless of style. If your nature is to pick something and stick with it, great. If your nature is to try different things, great. Some people are happy mastering the cooking of one meal, or one type of cuisine. Other people are happier trying many different recipes, each of which makes them a better cook overall, but they never master any single dish.

My meditation practice changes constantly. Sometimes I meditate in silence, sometimes with a background of white noise, or with music. Often, I will spend 40 minutes using one technique. Other times I will use three different techniques in a 15 minute meditation. The most important thing is just that you meditate, regardless of how. Establishing a regular practice can be hard for many people, so in the next chapter, we'll explore some of the tips for helping make this part of your daily life.

How Long to Meditate For?

This is a far more difficult question than it might seem. There are many answers. The teacher S.N. Goenka suggested you do two hours a day. MBSR prescribes forty-five minutes, six days a week. Transcendental Meditation suggests twenty minutes twice a day. They're different, but all good answers.

However, there is one important caveat before answering this question. It comes back to the point that habits are really hard to break. Whatever habit you start to develop with your practice will probably become permanent.

Imagine you have decided to get fit, strong, or lean. You make a commitment to go to the gym for one hour a day. But on your first visit, you are exhausted after ten minutes and decide to go to the juice bar to get refreshed. You sit down, and forty-five minutes go by. It's very nice. The next time you go to the gym you do the same thing. Very soon it's a habit.

I think meditation can be the same. You might be tempted to think, "I'm going to do an hour because I want what meditation offers." You start, and you might stay focused, and get distracted, and then refocused and distracted, and refocused and distracted for only five or ten minutes before you feel exhausted or frustrated and stop trying to refocus. If that happens, you will then spend the next fifty to fifty-five minutes merely thinking about your life, solving problems and daydreaming.

There's nothing wrong with thinking about your life, solving problems or daydreaming, but you want to try to avoid allowing yourself to slip into the habit of doing that while you're trying to meditate. This is tricky because your mind is going to think, to solve problems, and daydream when you're meditating, and that's fine. It's fine so long as every time you notice you are distracted you try to return your attention to the meditation.

If you start to sit in such a way that you are allowing your mind to go wherever it wants for long periods of time, that is going to be the habit you form with your practice, and it will be very hard for you to change that later. Start with short meditations, with high quality effort. The effort does not need to be one of strain, and please try to avoid judging yourself when you fail, but you want to develop the habit of diligent effort where you keep trying to return your focus to the meditation whenever you notice your attention has wandered. As you build meditation stamina, you can extend the time.

What is the optimal amount of time? The U.S. Army is keen to know the answer to this question. The Army currently loses more soldiers and ex-soldiers to suicide than they do as a result of enemy engagement. Meditation seems to be an effective tool to help. As a result, the Army is on board with giving their soldiers meditation training as part of the toolkit they need to be best equipped to deal with the trauma of war. But to take time to train troops in meditation is to take time away from other types of training. So they want to know what is the minimum amount of time you can meditate for the most benefit.

The neuroscientist Dr. Amishi Jha is at the forefront of this research and suggests the number is about twelve minutes a day. The early findings seem to suggest twelve is the number where you get the most benefit for the least amount of time spent. However, Jha herself has admitted that she prefers to do thirty. Twelve may be the sweet spot in terms of benefit received for time spent, but more is better.

Nevertheless, if you can only do five to start with, do five, and then build. Although twelve minutes might be the dose that delivers the greatest benefit for the time invested, five good minutes is worthwhile. When you start to see the benefits, you'll start to want to find longer periods of time to practice.

Some days I wake up late and have to get out the door to catch a plane, a train, or get to a meeting. For me, I like to get an hour a day, but sometimes five minutes is all I get. I'd still rather get five minutes in than none. Five minutes still makes a difference.

When is the Best Time to Meditate?

When you meditate – that's the best time to meditate. It is hard for most people who want to meditate every day to end up meditating every day. So whatever works for you, is good. Nevertheless, the general guideline is to try to do at least one meditation in the morning. It gets it done, it becomes part of your morning routine, and it sets your mind up for the day ahead. One tip I picked up from listening to Eileen Fisher (founder and CEO of the clothing company) suggested "Get up. Pee. Meditate." If you want to slip in getting a quick cup of tea or coffee to get you alert, that's okay too.

Your Phone

If you meditate first thing in the morning, try to avoid looking at your phone before you start. I know this is difficult for many people, and when you wake up, there is a powerful temptation to see what has happened in the world, who has sent us mail, or messages. If you possibly can, just leave it for a few more minutes. See if you can avoid engaging with all that information until after. Anything you read will act as fodder for your attention to start to process while you are trying to meditate. All that information will still be there after the meditation. It is unlikely that looking at it earlier will actually make a difference, but it will make it harder for you to hold your attention on the meditation.

One Session, or Multiple Sessions

Dividing your meditation up into multiple sessions, for example, the TM approach of twenty minutes twice a day does seem to be dramatically more beneficial than one forty-minute effort in the morning. But it can be hard enough to do one a day at first. You don't want to set yourself up for failure, which will discourage you. So start with seeing if you can get a good habit going of meditating once a day, and then see if you can incorporate a second one.

Can You Meditate Lying Down?

You can meditate standing up, walking, running, dancing, sitting in a chair, cross legged on the floor, or balancing in a headstand. Yes, you can also meditate lying down, but it is not advisable to try this first thing in the morning, or last thing at night. I'm sure everybody who has ever meditated tried at some point to do their morning meditation while still lying in bed. It doesn't work. You fall back to sleep. I'm sure you'll still try it. Don't judge yourself when you fail; you will not have been the first to think it was a good idea. Just don't believe that next time it'll work. Get your feet on the floor. Go pee. Maybe get a cup of tea or coffee. And then meditate.

CHAPTER EIGHT

Establishing a Practice

Many of my friends who meditate, don't meditate.

If you ask them if they meditate, they'll say yes. They are knowledgeable about meditation, are likely to tell you how wonderful it is, and will probably try to convince you that you should do it. They have a meditation cushion or bench. They might also have a special space set aside in their home with a small altar, a candle, and some incense sticks. Privately, however, they will admit that even with all that, and having the intention to meditate every day, they hardly ever get around to meditating. They want to meditate every day, and yet don't.

Meditation is not special in this way. For years I intended to go running every morning, but almost never did. I intended to write in my journal every day, but after a few days, I would stop. On many occasions, I have made a decision that I'm going to give up white carbohydrates. And sometime later that day I will cook a bowl of noodles. I've stopped bothering to set New Year's Resolutions for myself after realizing that my success rate with them is almost exactly the same as the rest of the population – somewhere very close to 0%.

I am not special. Almost everyone has difficulty with trying to create a new behavior, or with trying to stop an existing one. It is hard even if they have a powerful desire to change. It is challenging even when it is going to be beneficial for them to change, or harmful to them if they don't.

This is not a modern problem. Paul the apostle, who wrote much of Christianity's New Testament, complained in his letter to the Romans about "the good that I would, I do not: but the evil which I would not, that I do." He probably wasn't talking about choosing pizza instead of having a salad, but whatever his 'evil' was that he was doing, we can see that even a divinely inspired, so-called saint had problems getting himself to do what he knew he should be doing, and to stop doing what he knew he shouldn't.

A lack of information is rarely the problem. Take losing weight for example. It seems as though almost everyone wants to lose ten pounds (or for some of us a little more). Despite magazine covers constantly revealing the latest 'new' secret diet formula, we aren't suffering from not knowing how to lose the weight. Almost all diet programs can be summarized as eat less white carbs, more vegetables, and do some exercise. So we know what to do. But we don't do it.

Nor is the problem a lack of desire. The United States contributes more than any other country to alleviate starvation in the developing world. But domestically the U.S. spends even more than that on diet products. We are prepared to hand over lots of money for the latest South American herb that promises miraculous results; we join gyms that we don't go to. Even if we want to change our behavior, and we know what to do, we are not very good at doing it.

Powerful forces are at work trying to understand this problem. Public policy experts and health insurers are trying to get people to make healthier choices. Rehab for addiction is a huge and highly profitable business, so clinics are motivated to outdo each other with having the most successful outcomes. Advertising agencies and corporations want to know what it takes to make us change our routine choices in favor of their products. There has been a great deal of research done with some useful findings.

The Divided Self

We tend to think of ourselves primarily as rational beings. We see ourselves as the person who works, plays, has opinions, beliefs, likes, and dislikes. We tend to think of ourselves as being in control of our lives, our decisions, and our actions. However, it is perhaps helpful to see that from the ancient Greeks through to modern psychologists, most theories about who we are suggest the situation is more complicated. In many theories, our rational self is only one part of the puzzle, and most suggest it is the least powerful part of the puzzle.

In Plato's *Phaedrus* dialogue, Socrates describes the self as being like a chariot driver, holding the reins of two horses. One horse is honorable and well behaved and will try to go in one direction. The other is wild, temperamental and poorly behaved, often wanting to go in a different direction. Our struggle is that we have to get both horses to move in the same direction in order to go anywhere.

Sigmund Freud suggested the self was made up of its ego, superego, and id. It is like some combination of you as the adult (ego) trying to get an unruly child (your id) to do what you want it to do while being criticized by a judgmental parent figure behind you (superego).

Chip and Dan Heath propose a helpful model for understanding why change is hard, and how to achieve it. They simplify our divided self into having a rational mind, and an emotional mind. The rational mind is of the belief that we can change behavior by understanding a problem, devising a solution, and implementing it. For example, I eat too much and exercise too little; I will, therefore, eat less and exercise more. This model seems sensible enough, but needless to say it doesn't work terribly well. The Heath brothers suggest significant change does not happen based on ANALYZE-THINK-CHANGE, but rather it happens when the emotional self is engaged which requires more of a SEE-FEEL-CHANGE approach. We need to understand that unless the emotional mind is motivated towards the goal, and develops an emotional attachment to the outcome, and ideally also to the process, then change is unlikely to happen.

If you believe that meditating every day is a good idea, that's probably not going to be enough. If you have read about the benefits and you want those benefits, it probably isn't enough either. The rational self is not as powerful as the emotional self. I know from too many personal failures that having a good intention to get up early to meditate is not good enough. I have decided I want to meditate in the morning and set the alarm to get up early. On more mornings than I like to admit, I have hit the snooze button when the alarm went off and slept through my meditation time. That evening I would give myself a good talking to, remind myself of the reasons I want to meditate tomorrow, the alarm goes off, and I would hit snooze again.

The brutal truth is that if your rational mind wants to do something, but your emotional self wants to do something else, the emotional self will tend to win. So, you need your emotional self to want it, and this is not likely to be based on a rational evaluation of benefits. If you want to get up twenty minutes early to meditate, that has to be more attractive to your emotional mind than staying in bed for an extra twenty minutes – so it has to be pretty damned attractive.

For me, there have been a number of factors that have helped. I am not proud of any of them, but I am grateful for the result.

One has been to change the way I see meditating in the morning. I used to see it as a good idea. It was something I wanted to be doing. This was all very rational stuff. I changed that to see my choosing to meditate, or not, in terms of my happiness and unhappiness. I don't get up to meditate because it will make me happier because staying in bed an extra twenty minutes will also make me happier. I see not getting up as making a conscious decision, via my non-doing, to be more miserable. That hurts me. It feels stupid to make a decision to be more miserable. I have a powerful reaction to seeing myself as stupid. I *really* don't like feeling stupid. My emotional self doesn't like feeling that way. So, by seeing not-meditating in that way, I motivate myself to get out of bed.

Your Willpower Battery

Another piece of research I found helpful was around the concept of willpower by Roy Baumeister and his colleagues at Case Western Reserve University. They suggest that willpower is not a fixed resource within us where those who have it are somehow morally superior to those of us that don't. Our willpower is like a battery that starts full, but once it's used up, it no longer works. They measured the ability of students to resist temptation. In the first experiment, they offered students the option of cookies, carrots, and celery when the students hadn't eaten for a few hours. Most students went for the carrots and celery. However, in a separate version of the experiment, they started by getting the students to solve a number of complex problems. The students were given access to the solutions but asked to try not to look up the answers if they could avoid it. The students mostly resisted the temptation to cheat. But then they were given the same option of carrots and celery rather than cookies, and the results were completely different from the first group. Most students went for the sugary treat.

When you decide that you're going to get up 90 minutes early every day and start meditating, exercising, writing in your journal and eating more fruit, you are probably setting yourself up to fail. It will require a great deal of willpower that you may not have, and when you fail, you'll be discouraged. Taking on one change at a time is probably all you can manage.

The Power of Habits

If willpower is limited, your best chance of making a change stick is to stop needing willpower in the first place. Habits are things we do automatically, and willpower is not required. So how do you create a habit?

I regret there is no scientific basis for the widely held belief that if you do something for twenty-one days, twenty-eight days, or even thirty days that it becomes a habit. Research suggests the real number is somewhere higher than sixty days, and even then, it depends on how substantial the change is that you're making. What research has more helpfully discovered are some of the ways new habits get formed.

For one reason or another we make a choice one day to do something different. It might be taking a new route home, joining a colleague for a run, or trying some noodles when you're hungry. If there was a payoff of some kind, you are likely to do it again. If there was something negative to the new routine, you are unlikely to do it, regardless of the reasons you might have for trying again. Payoffs can be multifaceted, but in some way, it must make you happier, or diminish pain. Going a particular way home may cut out the risk of waiting at a long traffic light. Running might seem to be about getting exercise, but might also be about establishing a friendship with a new acquaintance. Cooking up noodles gives a quick carbohydrate hit with next to no effort.

At some point after this is repeated over and over, the reaction becomes automatic. You find yourself with no need to remember the journey home once you turn a particular corner. You and your friend just meet at the same place and same time every week. You're hungry, and you put the water on for noodles.

Once established, whether they are good or bad habits, they are very difficult to break. When I was trying to establish the habit of meditating every morning, I found it helpful to realize that I already had a habit in relation to meditation in the morning. I had a powerfully established habit of not meditating. Every day I didn't meditate I was reinforcing that habit, as opposed to creating a new one.

Another helpful aspect of habits that researchers look at is the nature of cues. The automatic response that is the habitual behavior has certain cues that trigger the response. For example, getting into your car and driving down a particular road triggers your automatic navigation of the new route, without needing to think about it. Seeing that it's Wednesday and six-thirty in the evening, means you need to go and get changed to meet your friend for a run. Hunger, as you walk into the kitchen, means you put the water on for the noodles. Understanding how this automaticity occurs is helpful in establishing new behavioral patterns or breaking old ones.

Whatever you have as your morning routine today is likely a series of habitual cues and reactions. Maybe the alarm goes off at 6.30am. You hit the snooze button for half an hour, get into the shower, get a cup of coffee and a piece of toast before heading out the door to work.

For me, I had a habit of waking up, feeling hungry and my automatic behavior became heading to the local shop to get a bagel and a cup of coffee. The payoff was delicious. The cue was just getting out of bed and feeling hungry. I would wake up, think about meditating, and then think "I'll meditate when I come back from coffee." Sometimes I would. Often, I wouldn't.

I realized I needed to change the cues and the payoffs. I made the bagel and coffee the payoff for meditating. I got up, threw some water on my face, made a cup of tea and sat down to meditate. Then, off for a bagel and coffee. I ended up looking forward to the meditation, partly for the meditation itself, but also so that I could then go and get breakfast.

The power of cues may be why many people find it easier to change patterns when on holiday or traveling. Waking up to a different bedroom, different alarm, different orientation of furniture prevents us from falling into the automatic behavior we have at home. We have to think about our morning ritual and decide what we want to do, what to wear, and how to get a cup of coffee.

To change your reaction to the cues in your current bedroom, try changing things around. Maybe change the orientation of your bed, or put your meditation cushion in front of the bathroom door before you go to sleep. You might try changing the alarm time to something odd and random, like 6:24 to trigger a different reaction, or change the default alarm from listening to a radio station to a new alert you've never used before.

AA

An unscientific but effective approach for changing behavior was established by Bill Wilson in the 1930s. Alcoholics Anonymous (AA) was the original twelve-step program whose success has spawned many similar programs that help people change destructive behaviors. It wasn't designed on the back of psychological research into alcohol addiction, but it has prospered because it works. Not 100% of the time by any means, but the twelve-step model remains one of the most effective programs for altering habitual behavior. Because of its success, researchers and psychologists have studied AA to try to understand why it works.

AA certainly recognizes the power of cues as triggers for unwanted behavior. Meeting friends in a bar, or seeing a bottle in the cupboard can trigger the automatic behavior that someone is trying to change. A lot of AA is about inviting people to understand their cues and to remove or avoid them as best as they can.

Another critical aspect of AA is the support of a community. At one level this seems obvious – having a support structure is useful. There is another part to this. One of our most basic needs as social creatures is to connect with others. Some experts on addiction even go so far as to suggest that many addictions are caused as a result of people's lack of connection to others. When someone joins an AA group, there is an immediate payoff by being with other individuals. This immediately starts to alleviate the original loneliness or alienation that may have first led them to drink or whatever other addiction they have.

There are now thousands of meditation groups around the world that get together daily, weekly, or monthly. A quick search on the Internet will give you lots of options. It can seem intimidating to just show up, but almost all groups will be welcoming and delighted to have another person, regardless of how much experience you have. If you don't like the first one you find, try another. They're all a little different.

You don't necessarily even need to join a group, you can just have some friends and agree to get together once a month to meditate. Maybe go out for dinner afterwards.

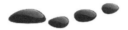

The research on changing behavior is still in its infancy and hopefully, will continue to deliver useful assistance in helping us make changes more easily in our lives. I've certainly found the research helpful in trying to establish my own habits. It helped to find an emotional connection to my meditation practice. I have set up cues that remind me to meditate. My practice is now a habit rather than something I need to will myself to do. I belong to several meditation communities, and at least once a week I meditate in a group.

Someone asked me recently if I meditated every day. I replied that I did. They said that was amazing, and that I must have great discipline. I was confused because I don't. I knew what they meant, but it occurred to me that it wasn't discipline that got me to where I am. I think I just never gave up trying to find a way to do it every day. If you've made it this far through this book, it means you have at least one of the most important attributes needed to establish a regular meditation practice – persistence.

If you have tried many times to establish a good routine, but it has not yet stuck, keep trying. On many occasions, my practice looked the same as that of my friends. I would say that I meditated, but I wasn't really meditating. There were long periods of good, steady, regular practice, and long periods of nothing. I tried many different tactics and strategies for getting my habit going. I'm not certain what single thing ended up making the difference, except that I kept trying. I encourage you to do the same. Don't give up. There's so much on offer from meditation, so stick with it. Try some of the suggestions from the research. Stay creative. Keep looking at the problem in new ways and try new solutions. Join or form a community. At some point, the pieces will align, and you will find yourself doing it every day, without needing discipline or willpower, enjoying everything meditation has to offer.

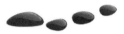

May you be happy. May you be healthy. May your life be filled with joy.

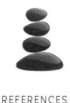

References

I've tried to keep this book as reference free as possible, focusing on my experiences and what I've observed. But, on occasion, I have broken my rule. Here is some explanation of some of the references I've used.

INTRODUCTION

- I've heard different variations of the story of the man on the horse but found this version in *The Heart of the Buddha's Teaching: Transforming Suffering into Peace, Joy, and Liberation,* Thich Nhat Hanh, 2015.

CHAPTER 1 – What is Meditation?

- There are many Transcendental Meditation centers around the world. Their main website is **tm.org**. The David Lynch Foundation is also an excellent charity that teaches TM with less of a religious context – **davidlynchfoundation.org**.

- The stimulus and response quote is from Viktor Frankl's *Man's Search for Meaning* which was first published in 1959.

- MBSR or Mindfulness Based Stress Reduction was founded by Jon Kabat-Zinn at UMass Medical Center in 1979. The main eight-week program is offered all around the world and online. **http://umassmed.edu/cfm/mindfulness-based-programs**

- If you want a great tour around Burgundy, you can find Florian at Bourgogne Evasion – **burgundybiketour.com**.

CHAPTER 2 – Relationships
PART ONE: Making Connection

- *You Can't Always Get What You Want*, from Let It Bleed, The Rolling Stones, 1969.

CHAPTER 4 – The Pursuit of Happiness

- I took the story of Martin Seligman and his daughter from *Authentic Happiness*, Martin Seligman, 2002. His follow up *Flourish* is even better as a presentation of Positive Psychology.

- Matt Killingsworth and Dan Gilbert's "A Wandering Mind Is an Unhappy Mind" was published in Science Magazine in November 2010. The research continues at **trackyourhappiness.org** where you can download an updated version of the app they used for the original study.

- "America's State of Mind," was the title of the 2011 Medco Report.

CHAPTER 5 - Health

- The comment about wild animals not getting diseases is a tacit reference to Robert M. Sapolsky's *Why Zebras Don't Get Ulcers*, 1994, W.H. Freeman.

- Kabat-Zinn talks about the irony of breathing being the best part of the MBSR program in *Full Catastrophe Living: using the wisdom of your body and mind to face stress, pain, and illness*, 1991.

- Blackburn and Epel's research into meditation and telomerase was presented in the journal Psychoneuroendocrinology as "Intensive meditation training, immune cell telomerase activity, and psychological mediators." However, if scientific research papers aren't your thing, they also present their larger body of research in their co-authored book, *The Telomere Effect: A Revolutionary Approach to Living Younger, Healthier, Longer*, 2017.

CHAPTER 7 – How to Meditate

- Dr. Jha's work can be found at **www.amishi.com**. This reference to the twelve-minute optimal meditation came from an interview Dan Harris did with her and Major General Walter Platt as part of the 10% Happier Podcast series in 2016.

- "Get up. Pee. Meditate." This also came from Dan Harris's excellent 10% Happier Podcast series when he interviewed Eileen Fisher in 2016.

CHAPTER 8 – Establishing a Practice

- The St Paul quote is from his letter to the Romans, Chapter 7, verse 19.

- I have taken the research on habits and changing behavior from several sources, including

  - *Switch: How to Change Things When Change is Hard*, Chip and Dan Heath, 2010.

  - *Willpower: Rediscovering the Greatest Human Strength*, Roy Baumeister, 2012.

  - *Making Habits, Breaking Habits*, Jeremy Dean, 2013.

  - *The Power of Habit*, Charles Duhigg, 2014.

Acknowledgements

Primarily I owe thanks to all my teachers for what they have shown me. I am forever in their debt. Some, in the early days especially, were sowing seeds without me even realizing it, and I regret I can only remember the moments, I cannot remember their names. I am sorry, and nonetheless grateful. Some of these that I can name worked with me for years, some only in passing. Most are still alive, but sadly some are not. Thank you all: Ananda, Jim Bonney, John Bowker, Judson Brewer, Brother Michael, Gangaji, Stephan Harker, Mr Hicks, Stan Koehler, Julius Lipner, Chris Lloyd, Mark Loughridge, Chris O'Neill, Rama, Saki Santorelli, Sogyal Rinpoche, RyuShin, and Carolyn West.

Thank you to the early readers of the manuscript, many of whom have been my cheerleaders, keeping me going throughout this process. It is far better thanks to all of you: Reed Alpert, Janet Broderick, Andy Huchingson, Douglas Martin, Juliet McGhie, Bailey Meadows, Rhea, Dominic Streatfeild-James, Mike Wallace, Diana Flaminzeanu. Special thanks go to David Comer – for being a great Dad, a terrific editor, and also for being okay with me keeping the piece about his parenting.

Mindy Gibbins-Klein of The Book Midwife - thank you. Another successful delivery of which I hope you are proud.

Thank you also to my fellow Book Midwife authors who have helped me along the journey and kept me inspired by your courage and determination: Angela, Elva, Hazel, Karen, Kate, Mary, and Zara.

And Sally. I've often thought it was trite when authors thanked their partners, wives, or families. It seemed as though they were just using it as a way to get some credit in the relationship bank after spending too much time on their own writing away. Now I understand it is real. I knew writing this would be hard; it was just harder than I expected. Sally helped me when the writing was good, and when it was bad, when I was inspired, and when I was demoralized. Without her continued and unconditional support, this would never have come into being. Thank you with all my heart.

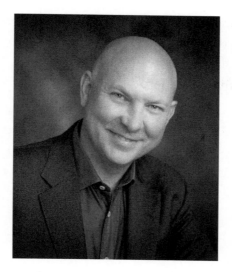

About the Author

Justyn Comer has been practicing meditation for over thirty years and teaching since 1999. He is a co-founder of RWM Education, Inc., a non-profit organization dedicated to making meditation available to as many people as possible. More information is available at www.realworldmeditation.org.

All royalties from the sale of this book will go to RWM Education, Inc.